Catwalk looks

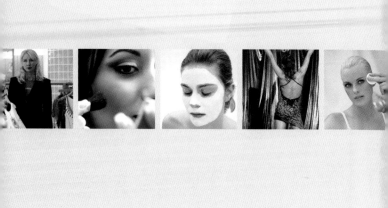

Catwalk **looks**

52 brilliant little ideas to
lose weight and stay slim

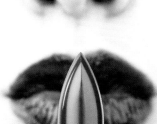

Linda Bird & Cherry Maslen

brilliantideas

CAREFUL NOW

Follow the tips in this book and you should find yourself looking at a fitter, sexier more glamorous you in the mirror. However, while you can transform yourself into the most gorgeous you you've ever been don't expect to become Elle McPherson overnight. The tips in this book are tried and tested – but you'll have to work at it (like all the rest of us) if you want results. Now get out there and start turning heads.

Infinite Ideas would like to thank Linda Bird, Eve Cameron, Kate Cook, Peter Cross, Helena Frith Powell, Lisa Helmanis, Lynn Huggins-Cooper, Cherry Maslen, Lizzie O'Prey, Marcelle Perks, Steve Shipside and Elisabeth Wilson for their contributions to this book.

First published in 2006 by
The Infinite Ideas Company Limited
36 St Giles
Oxford, OX1 3LD
United Kingdom
www.infideas.com

A CIP catalogue record for this book is available from the British Library

ISBN 13: 978-1-904902-32-4
ISBN 10: 1-904902-32-4

Brand and product names are trademarks or registered trademarks of their respective owners.

Designed and typeset by Baseline Arts Ltd, Oxford
Printed in Singapore

Brilliant ideas

Introduction

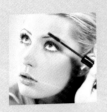

We need to start this introduction with an apology. Unless you are called Gisele, Heidi, Cindy or Naomi there's very little chance that you'll be parading around on a catwalk any time soon.

Having said that, the little ideas in this book can help you make the very best of your natural assets and help you look and feel your most gorgeous every time you leave the house.

We all have aspects of our appearance we sometimes feel dissatisfied with and in most cases all we're missing out on are a few simple tips and tricks to take our appearance to the next level. Whether you want to lose the frizz from your hair, smooth the bumps in your bum cheeks, find the perfect bikini, sort out your personal style or just look younger and perkier, it's all covered in our quick to read and easy to implement ideas.

You might think you need a bit more than a bit of exercise and the perfect lipstick in order to look your best, so we've also taken a look at some of the more involved methods of beautification. Read on for the low-down on the latest salon treatments, the truth about expensive beauty products (do they really work?) and even the inside track on cosmetic surgery.

Taking care of your appearance doesn't mean you're shallow or vain but neither should it be the be-all and end-all of your life. Somebody who worries constantly about her appearance is never going to be attractive, no matter how many beauty products she applies, hours she spends in the gym or designer outfits she owns.

The biggest tip for being attractive is to go out there and enjoy yourself – and who cares if a few hairs are out of place.

1. Look great in photos

Adopt these clever postures and easy make-up techniques and the camera _will_ lie when you want it to.

Next time you have to face your public, try some of the following tricks picked up from the stars and the photographers.

- Try standing with one foot slightly in front of the other and gently pivot on your feet so that your body, including your shoulders, is at a slight angle to look slimmer. Putting your hands on your hips can make your waist look smaller. If you're sitting down, lean forward and rest your elbows on your knees to disguise wobbly thighs and look slimmer.

- Look lively: some professional portrait photographers insist the best pictures are always taken when the subject is looking animated and chipper. That way the subject's personality is captured. You can still engineer your 'best side' in front of the camera.

Here's an idea for you...

Maximise your lips. To pout beautifully, turn to the camera and say 'Wogan'. Bizarre, I know, but glamour models swear by it.

Defining idea

'With charm you've got to get up close to see it; style slaps you in the face.'

JOHN COOPER CLARKE, poet and comedian

- Practise in front of the mirror like you're bound to have done as a teenager. Perfect a pose you're happy with so you can strike it the moment the camera comes out.

- Brighten up: black can drain the colour from the face so choose brighter colours for your top half to bring out the best in your skin tone. However, beware of brightly patterned clothes, which can swamp you and detract from your face.

- Dark circles or bags under your eyes? Try lifting your chin to avoid shadows falling on your face.

- Everyone looks more attractive when they're looking happy and a lovely smile really does take the focus away from the bits you're less happy with.

- Putting your hair up can soften your features and draw attention to your smile.

- Get the photographer to take more than one photo! The more you have taken, the more likely it is you'll be captured from a flattering angle.

- Be subtle with make-up. Overdo the slap and you'll look like a waxwork or, worse, a cross-dresser. Apply a light foundation only where necessary, such as to the sides of your nose or over spots. To avoid a shiny face, stick to matt-formula make-up for your blemishes and only use creamy, reflective concealers for your eyes. Don't forget the golden rule of make-up though: never overplay both eyes and lips.

■ Flatter your best features. Apply blush over the apple part of your cheeks, sneak a couple of extra false lashes on your eyelids and slick on some glossy lipstick.

■ Ask for a minute or two before the camera clicks so you can touch up and dab a bit of powder over any shiny bits.

2. The confidence factor

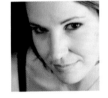

The trick to being sexy is to believe in and accept yourself.

Sex appeal is not just skin deep, it's also a question of attitude. Confident people are magnetic and captivating but not necessarily drop-dead gorgeous. These are usually people who are open, gregarious, amusing and positive. All attributes which require confidence.

Here's an idea for you...

Write down the five things (not necessarily physical) that most attract you to someone. And then work out how you can adapt them to work for you. Practise these small things and you'll already feel sexier and more confident.

15

Defining idea

'No one can make you feel inferior without your consent.'
ELEANOR ROOSEVELT

Set yourself small, achievable goals every week, and use them to boost your self esteem. Everyone has bad days but try to look at yourself like a stock. Your share price will go up or down, depending on market perception. If things are going well, and you're on a high, your stock will soar; everyone wants to know you. If you're at a low then your price will drop. And you won't help this drop in price by moping around refusing to go out. You need to work at it until your share price is right up there again. A new haircut, a new outfit, a new career move, anything that will boost you over the bad period. So here are my top six tips for becoming more confident or feigning confidence:

1. Think about your good points and accentuate them. For example, if you have lovely eyes, use them when you're talking to people or flirting.
2. DO NOT think about your bad points. You may think the spot just under your chin is the most dramatically dreadful thing to happen to you all year but chances are no one has even noticed it.
3. Feel good, look good. Be healthy. Eat well and exercise. If you feel like you're in shape, you will ooze confidence.
4. A new outfit/haircut/lip gloss can do wonders for your confidence levels. Treat yourself before an important date.

5. It's not about what you've got but what people think you've got. So if you feel your chest is a tad too flat, invest in a Wonderbra. If your lips are not plump enough then use some lip-liner to accentuate them.
6. Remain slightly mysterious. Fantasy is often better than reality. Don't give too much away.

If you feel suddenly insignificant then cast your mind back to your vast list of achievements and plus points. And remember, the person you're talking to is probably not as confident as they are pretending to be either…

3. Hands-on treatments

Your hands speak volumes. Fortunately, if you can't stretch to salon manicures, there are easy ways to titivate your nails on the cheap.

Your hands *do* get noticed and a neatly manicured pair say you're well-groomed and glamorous.

Here's an idea for you...

A nightly trick to soften hands is to smother Vaseline or petroleum jelly into your nails, which will have a dramatic effect on taming your cuticles. For best results wear gloves to bed afterwards and you'll wake with beautifully soft hands.

The first step to gorgeous hands is to wash and dry them regularly and to always use hand cream. Keep a jar by every sink in your house plus one in your handbag. However, as crucial as washing your hands may be, it pays to minimise the time your hands spend submerged in water so always use rubber gloves when washing up and when cleaning as household-cleaning products can make your skin dry and your nails dry and brittle.

Eat your way to better nails. The best foods for nails include plenty of protein (fish, meat, soya, tofu, eggs) to help them grow and prevent those white lines from appearing. B vitamins found in eggs, seafood and root vegetables are a good way to keep those nasty ridges at bay. Eat plenty of fish, fish oils and seeds, which are all rich in essential fatty acids that help nourish nails, as well as foods rich in zinc, such as seafood, lean meat and wholegrains, to help prevent white spots. Brittle nails? You'll need to eat lots of calcium and vitamin-A foods such as carrots, peaches, leafy vegetables and tinned fish, which are great for strengthening dry nails.

Treat yourself to a home manicure every week or two and save the real thing for special occasions. Remove old polish and then shape each nail with an emery board (nail files are too severe). Don't saw away at your nails or you'll break them. Instead, use light strokes from the edges towards the centre. Massage your cuticles with cuticle cream or add a few drops of cuticle massage oil to a bowl of warm water. Soak your

Defining idea

'Without grace, beauty is an unbaited hook.'
FRENCH PROVERB

cuticles for five minutes, then push them back using a cuticle stick. Wash your hands, then apply a protective base coat of clear varnish to your nails, then a coat or two of colour. Leave your hands for twenty minutes or so to avoid smudging them, then add a sealing topcoat.

Don't forget to apply sunscreen to your hands. We rarely think about protecting our hands from the sun because we rarely burn there, but hands will give away your age better than any other part of your body and can even add a few cruel years too, so look after them.

4. Beans means lines

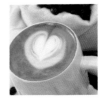

Caffeine can make cellulite worse so if you're a coffee fiend, it's time to switch to decaf. Here's why.

■ Caffeine can contribute to weight gain. Drinking two cups of coffee is enough to raise the levels of the stress hormone cortisol and insulin in your body, which is thought to accelerate ageing and encourage the body to store fat. It also makes us more likely to be tempted by sugary treats. When coffee drinkers reduce their coffee intake, they lose weight.

- Caffeine is also bad for your skin because it impedes your blood circulation and oxygenation, leading to dark circles, puffiness, fine lines, poor colour. The skin on your behind is going to look dry and dehydrated, making the cellulite worse.

- Caffeine is a diuretic and can dehydrate your body. When you're dehydrated, cells hold on to water – and your fat cells hold on to fluids, which, on your bottom and thighs, make your skin bulge out and look puffier and more dimply.

- Caffeine can worsen symptons of PMS. Coffee also causes your body to get rid of important nutrients, especially B vitamins, which are needed for energy, good skin and hair, healthy growth, and mood.

- Caffeine destroys calcium – one cup of coffee destroys about 6mg of calcium from your body's stores. Experts have found that calcium is important in weight loss because it's thought to help prevent fat storage and boost metabolism.

Defining idea

'Behind every successful woman is a substantial amount of coffee.'
STEPHANIE PIRO, artist

So how much is too much? About 300 mg caffeine a day is 'a moderate' intake. One cup of coffee contains about 100 mg per 190ml, tea 30–60 mg per 190ml cup and cola

around 50 mg per can.
So 4 cups of tea or one cup of coffee would give you roughly half of your 'allowance'. Chocolate also contains caffeine; in fact there's about 10 mg of caffeine in 50 g of milk chocolate – dark chocolate contains 28 mg per 50 g (not to mention the fat content).

Here's an idea for you...

Ditch that coffee and start your day with a large glass of freshly squeezed orange juice and a bowl of berries. They're packed with vitamin C, which is important for the production of collagen and can strengthen the capillaries, which feed the skin. And better skin can mean smoother thighs.

Best advice, then, is to cut down as much as you can – don't drink more than one or two cups of coffee a day – and look instead for healthy alternatives.

5. Work it!

You have to be smart and sassy at 8am and gorgeous and sexy at 8pm and there is no time to go home in between.

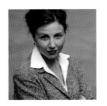

Start your preparation the night before. Go to bed early, having had a long bath, done your nails, waxed your legs, plucked your eyebrows and so forth. Get into bed wearing a moisturising mask – believe me it's worth the messy pillowcase in the morning.

Here's an idea for you...

Take another pair of shoes to the office to change into for the evening. There's nothing quite as refreshing as taking off shoes you have been running around in all day.

Next morning, have a shower, wash your hair and prepare yourself as you normally would for a day at work. The time between leaving work and the date needs to be used to give you that 'just left the bathroom' look. To achieve this you will have to bring to the office make-up remover, moisturiser, toothbrush, hairbrush, scent, deodorant, new underwear, tights/stockings and a change of clothes. If a complete new outfit sounds too much then a glamorous evening top and shoes to twin with your day wear can transform your outfit.

Once you have finished your high-powered day, lock yourself in the lady's loo. If the one at the office isn't very nice then be bold: walk to the nearest luxury hotel and march into theirs. If you walk in looking confident people rarely question you.

Once in a bathroom, remove day make-up and immediately apply your moisturiser. Then wash under your arms (it's amazing how much fresher you will feel if you do this); if you can, also wash your feet. People may come in wondering what on earth you're on, but if you want to smell and look good for your special night out do you

really care if you end up with a
reputation for being a bit quirky?

Defining idea

'Be prepared.'
MOTTO OF THE SCOUT ASSOCIATION

Once you're washed, brush your
teeth, change your clothes, then
apply your make-up, brush your hair, spray on some scent and
you're ready. If you have about half an hour and your date is in a
town or city, you might want to nip into a hairdresser's for a quick
wash and blow dry. Then you can do your make-up there. But you
should probably get the underarm and feet washing out of the way
beforehand!

Now you look ready for your night out just give yourself a few
minutes to shake away the mental stresses of work and get into
party mode and the transformation is complete.

6. Move that body

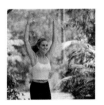

**Exercise has the potential to transform
your body and do wonders for your skin.**

Exercise makes you feel great, is great for your
complexion and keeps you looking younger.
The good news is that even a small amount of exercise can make a

Here's an idea for you...

Fidgeting can burn up to 800 calories a day. So turn sitting at your desk, driving or an evening vegging in front of the TV into a workout. Make a point of shifting around every fifteen minutes – adjust your posture, roll your shoulders or change the way you cross your legs.

major difference.

Increasing oxygen to the skin boosts your complexion. At rest the average person takes in about 0.5 litres of air with every breath, but with exercise your air intake can increase to 4.5 litres per breath, which means a lot more oxygen is getting to your skin.

Experts say we should aim for a minimum of three twenty- to thirty-minute aerobic sessions per week, such as running, swimming, cycling, dancing or brisk walking. If possible, also try to add in three half-hour sessions of weight or resistance work, which increases muscle mass and can boost our body's metabolism and improve the way our body handles free radicals that wreak havoc on our body, including our skin – invest in some dumbbells or try walking or cycling uphill.

Start small and be realistic about what you want to achieve. Every week aim to do something, even if it's a twenty-minute stroll every other day. Make a list of what you're going to do each week and stick to it. And try to change your approach to exercise. If you think in terms of activities rather than workouts and 'burning calories' it will sound less like a chore. Swimming, hiking, cycling, walking or rollerblading are far more appealing than going to the gym. They're fun, burn calories and are great for sculpting thighs, bottoms and legs.

If you make a social event of your exercise, you're more likely to stick at it. In one recent study, people who made friends at their gym tended to exercise more often than

people without gym buddies. If you're not a gym member, make dates to walk or exercise with a friend to help you keep on track.

If you build up to a variety of different forms of exercise each week you're less likely to get bored, and you'll tone up different parts of your body. So try swimming (burns almost 200 calories in half an hour), then power-walking (300 calories in half an hour), plus have an exercise-video session or do a few sets of press-ups – great for a toned bust. Yoga is a great way to firm up your flabby bits and wipe the stress from your face.

7. Slimming treatments

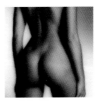

Lotions, potions and treatments promise all kinds of miracles. But are they worth the money?

To lose weight, you have to watch what you eat as well as spending money on some gimmicky product. The cosmetics industry will produce clinical studies proving that X cream really does help you lose inches, refine your silhouette or firm your curves, while most other doctors and scientists will say that what you apply from the outside doesn't make a blind bit of difference. So it can be hard to find out how effective these products really are.

Some of these treatments may well have an effect, though it's probably short-lived. Don't underestimate the psychological element – there's no doubt that looking after yourself does make you feel good, which can spur you on to losing weight. Here's our lowdown on some of the most readily available products and treatments.

Salon treatments

These usually involve being massaged, wrapped or painlessly zapped with some sort of electrical current. Massage is undoubtedly soothing and is claimed to stimulate your lymphatic system, which drains waste fluid from your tissues. You'll feel good afterwards, but not thinner. Wraps can shrink inches, but it's just fluid loss – they are fab for feeling a bit thinner for a special occasion. Electrical impulses stimulate your muscles by working them while you lie back and read a magazine. You would see better results with regular exercise.

Here's an idea for you...

A fake tan can make you look slimmer and leaner by sculpting, shadowing and highlighting muscles and curves. For the best results, have it applied in a salon. It will usually last for about five days.

Fat-busting creams

Despite the claims, you really won't get results unless you eat less and move more too. Still, they do make your skin feel very smooth and soft and strokable.

Colonic irrigation

This is based on the principle that toxic deposits are stored in your large intestine. When these are flushed out, it kickstarts the metabolism and helps elimination. If having a speculum inserted in your anus and having gallons of water sloshing around your insides is your idea of a good time, go right ahead! While many alternative practitioners say it's perfectly safe and even emotionally rewarding, conventional doctors reject the idea, some even saying it's downright dangerous.

Defining idea

After forty a woman has to choose between losing her figure or her face. My advice is to keep your face and stay sitting down.'
BARBARA CARTLAND

8. Keep an eye on your eyebrows

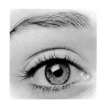

Eyebrows can take years off you if you shape them right. Here's how

Trim, neat, naturally ascending arched brows can make your eyes appear much bigger and give you a more youthful appearance. If yours are wild and tousled, you're missing a key beauty trick.

If you're going to splurge on a visit to the beautician, some would say that eyebrow shaping is *the* treatment to have done. It doesn't cost the earth, but it's a fabulous investment and you can then have your brows shaped just two or three times yearly as you'll have a template to follow whereby you can simply 'tidy' them once or twice a week with a pair of tweezers.

Home plucking: the rules

You can make some pretty awful mistakes with eyebrows and end up looking permanently surprised, shifty or indeed botoxed to within an inch of your life. Always pluck in a good light and invest in a magnifying mirror so things are much clearer.

- Start by brushing your eyebrows, using an eyebrow brush or small, soft toothbrush. Then trim any long hairs with nail scissors.
- Aim for a natural gently curving arch, thicker in the inner corner of the eye and tapering out over your brow bone. Focus on accentuating this natural curve by tidying up around it, above (forget that old myth, you *can* pluck above the brow) and below.
- Each eyebrow should start directly above the corner of the eye. Hold a pencil vertically along the side of your nose and remove any wild or stray hairs on the bridge of your nose beyond the pencil with a pair of tweezers. To see where your eyebrow should end, hold the pencil diagonally from your nostril to the end of your eye and pluck anything below the pencil to open up your eyes and to avoid looking droopy and drowsy.
- Work on the natural arch. To find the highest part of the arch,

keep your eye on the outer edge of your iris. Tweeze any hairs underneath that arch. Don't go mad though, as natural is always better.

For a fuller look, try brushing your brows sideways with your little toothbrush or eyebrow brush. Or slick them down using Vaseline or a bit of moisturiser, no need for expensive eyebrow gel. Slicked eyebrows do make you look instantly groomed, so it's worth experimenting.

Here's an idea for you...

Give yourself a facial workout to help tone your facial muscles. Stand in front of the mirror daily and raise your eyebrows as high as possible and simultaneously open your eyes as wide as you can. Slowly lower your eyebrows and relax. Repeat this five times.

9. Dressed to kill

Whether it's fancy dress or a formal affair, what should you wear?

There is nothing worse than arriving at an event and realising that you have chosen completely the wrong outfit. If you turn up in a little black dress and gorgeous jewels and everyone else has shown up in jeans, then it takes a great deal of composure to carry off the outfit without embarrassment. And of course the same is true of the reverse situation.

Defining idea

'Elegance is innate...It has nothing to do with being well-dressed.'
DIANA VREELAND

Chances are that the dress code will be indicated on the invitation. Black tie means formal dress and white tie means long gowns, not cocktail dresses. Check with one or two fellow invitees to find out what they are going to wear so that you can gauge the style of your outfit accordingly. Make sure you feel happy and confident in what you are wearing. Don't vamp up your style of dress if that's not the kind of person that you are.

It is particularly important at weddings that you do not wear anything that will detract or take the focus away from the bride. Bear in mind that you are probably going to be photographed with the couple. You do not want the bride to be disappointed with her wedding album just because your outfit stands out in every picture.

Fancy dress

If you are going to ask people to dress up, make sure that everyone who is invited knows about it – and make sure that they know that coming in 'normal' party clothes is unacceptable. There is nothing worse than donning an outrageous outfit and walking into a room where most of the other people haven't 'turned out'. As a guest, the best way to avoid this happening is to go and hire outfits with a group of friends so that you know there'll be safety in numbers.

It is easier for people to decide what to wear if you give your fancy dress party a theme. Heroes and Villains is always a good one and Nursery Rhymes provides plenty of scope if there are going to be children at the party too.

Whatever the choice, party gear or fancy dress, plan your outfit well in advance to avoid last minute panics and the possibility that 'you don't have anything to wear'!

Here's an idea for you...

Pick a style that suits your build. If you are short or have a full figure, you might consider something 'empire line', which, with the seam just under the bust, means that the flowing fabric below is complementary to your shape. If you are tall and slim then a long, form-fitting dress can look stunning. Chubby arms look best in long loose sleeves; if you are quite bony, opt for fitted three-quarter length sleeves.

10. The blushing bride

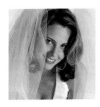

It's a must to be realistic when searching for the right wedding dress.

Your wedding dress is unlike any dress you will ever have worn. So throw away your preconceptions of what will suit you: you'll be wrong. Try on every shape you can get your hands on, even if you

Defining idea

'Clothes make the man. Naked people have little or no influence on society.'
MARK TWAIN

don't like the style. You are guaranteed to be surprised by what flatters you. And that goes for your complexion, too: pure white doesn't work for everyone so make sure you see the dress against your skin in daylight as well as in the shop, because your guests will.

When you have found a style that suits, compare the cost of materials. This will give you an idea of what you need to consider when setting your budget. Now you can look at the wedding magazines, to help you find variations on your theme. You will need to order at least three to four months before your big day and, if you are indecisive, work back from this date to make sure you don't end up panic buying.

You need a dress buddy to talk you out of any childish Cinderella fantasy, and give her free rein to say, 'Yes, your bum does look big in that'. Try on the dress with the height of heel you intend to wear. Having your dress cut a few inches too short could be devastating, sartorially speaking.

Think about the season of your wedding. High summer fabrics include cool silk, chiffon, pure cotton or lace while cooler winter months call for heavier fabrics such as brocade, velvet and duchess satin. And be practical: hiking a huge skirt through fields to a marquee might seem funny at first but will soon lose its humorous appeal.

Write a list of all your best assets and those which you would like to show off to full advantage on the day. A lovely off-the-shoulder number is ideal for a long neck, and a pear shape can be hidden with a slinky waist, flaunting a full skirt and nipped-in bodice. You will

Here's an idea for you...

When choosing your dress, think first about your hairstyle and headdress, or absence of one. Different necklines will work better with hair up or down, with veil or without.

never have a chance to hide your disliked bits so skilfully again! And don't forget that budgets often get stretched by essentials such as underwear, stockings, shoes, jewellery, bags, scarves, etc. All will add finishing touches and complete your look, but will they bust your budget?

11. Lose 10lbs without dieting

Dress cleverly – in shades, cuts and styles to suit you. It's the simplest way to a slimmer and more shapely you.

Dark colours certainly can minimise the bulges, but it's not the only sartorial route to a more slender you. Instead, be inventive and follow these guidelines.

Defining idea

'I have always said that the best clothes are invisible... They make you notice the person.'
KATHARINE HAMNETT

- Create the illusion of being longer and leaner by dressing head to foot in the same shade, even white.
- Don't buy the snug size ten just because that's your usual size. You can lose pounds by wearing slightly looser clothes that skim over bumps and hang flatteringly.
- Lined clothes won't hug you so unforgivingly. Lined trousers are a godsend, particularly in summer, as they drop crisply, however hot and sweaty you are beneath.
- A-line skirts flatter almost everyone because they don't cling to your curves and do minimise your bottom. The best length is on or just below the knee and if you team it with knee-length boots you can disguise thick legs and hefty unfeminine thighs. In the summer, a light-coloured skirt can look great with suede boots.
- Hipster jeans can be really flattering as they create the illusion of having smaller hips. Keep a close eye on the flesh overhang, however, which can ruin the effect, and stick to the boot-leg cut, which is flattering as it makes your legs look longer and slimmer.
- Always wear a heel, however tall you are. The extra inch or two will add length and can make you more aware of your posture.
- Stick to textured fabrics, which can help to 'break up' flesh.
- Disguise a big bust with V-necks and low scoop necks. Slash necks and halter necks will make you look bulky.

- Always choose trousers with hems long enough to skim the tip of a boot or shoe. This will immediately draw the eye down, giving the impression of a longer, leaner leg. Avoid tapered trousers, clam diggers and pedal pushers, which make almost everyone's thighs look bigger and legs look shorter and squatter than they are.

- Go for well-fitting bras with uplift and knickers that flatten in the right places. With bras, aim to banish seams, puckering and surplus flesh bursting out of cups.

Here's an idea for you...

Colour experts say white, silver and mother of pearl are 'eternally feminine'. Investing in striking silver or pearl jewellery is the easiest way to wear these colours. A soft shell-pink wrap and mother-of-pearl make-up will look particularly great against a tan. Light colours close to your face can reflect light and take years off you, too.

12. The power of lovely lingerie

Get your underwear right and you'll feel and look great.

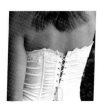

There are days when your cotton no-frills knickers work well. But to feel (and therefore look) truly glamorous you can't beat a matching bra and knickers set. For this reason you should seriously consider buying at least two pairs of knickers with each bra. To make sure you don't suffer from the dreaded VPL under trousers always make at least one of these pairs a G-string, or try out French knickers or boxer shorts for girls.

There is nothing like good underwear to enhance your body shape and make you feel more attractive. For the flatter-chested among us, there is no more comforting moment than pulling a T-shirt over a new Wonderbra and seeing our body shapes totally transformed. For larger ladies, a good well-fitting bra is even more essential. If you want to minimise your bust under business suits, get measured by an expert to find out your correct cup size – you will lose 10lbs, I swear, immediately you put on the right fitting bra. And if you want to emphasise your cleavage, a right fitting bra does this stupendously well, besides being much more comfortable.

If you're wearing the right underwear, you feel like you can take on the world. It makes you feel so much more confident. You walk into a business meeting and although the others can't see what you've got on underneath your suit, you know, and it gives you a sense of superiority.

As we all know, for whatever reason, men *adore* stockings and suspenders. They can also make you feel more powerful and sexy. Our job here is not to analyse, just wear them. Classic black suspender belts are the best but red can be good for a special occasion, adding an extra sex-vixen allure. The great thing about glamorous or sexy underwear is that it enhances your sex drive as well as your partner's. You're hardly going to sit around feeling like a drudge in a fabulous ensemble made of luxurious silk and lace.

13. Luscious lips

If you don't possess plump, bee-stung, kissable lips, you may want a few tips on how to fake them.

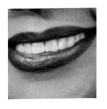

Size is a good starting point. You can minimise a large mouth and lips that are too full by choosing a neutral tone of lipstick. Use a lipliner to draw a line just inside the lips and choose a dark shade of lipstick to fill, which will help to make them look smaller. Therefore stay clear of dark colours if your lips are thin, as they'll make them look even smaller. Instead, use a lipliner to draw a line just over your

Here's an idea for you...

Go for berries, plums and blue-based red lipsticks, where the contrast will help make your teeth appear whiter and brighter. Avoid any yellow- or orange-based shades, including corals and browny colours, because they can make your teeth look yellow.

natural lip line to create the illusion of fuller lips and then go for a bright colour to plump them up more. Glossy or pearl lipsticks can also make lips look fuller, as they reflect the light.

Select the right shade of lippy. Finding the right colour is essential. Experts say that olive skins look their best next to berry shades. If your complexion and hair are fair, stick to reds with pinkish undertones. If you have pale skin and dark hair you'll find that strong, bright-red lipstick can look amazing. And if your skin is dark, then pick deep, rich reds.

Pay your lips due attention. Take the time to care for your lips in the same way that you care for your skin. Gently buff them with a soft, baby's toothbrush to remove dry skin and boost the circulation, then regularly apply lip balm. This is also a great way to soften up dry, cracked lips.

Try the bee-stung look. There's an art to perfecting bee-stung lips, but even those of us with thin lips can pout with the best of them. Try this:

- First, outline your lips using a lip pencil in the same shade as your lipstick or lighter (never darker, unless you're a lap dancer or would like to be mistaken for one).

Defining idea

'Beauty, to me, is about being comfortable in your own skin. That, or a kick-ass red lipstick.'
GWYNETH PALTROW

- Then, using a lip brush, 'fill in' your lips. Instead of using a block of matt colour, build up gradually using a sheer lipstick. That way you'll capture the light, which will make your lips look fuller and plumper.

- Using a highlighter pen, draw a fine line around your upper lips, just above your Cupid's bow. Alternatively, try blending little dots of reflective foundation on your upper lips, which will also help accentuate a natural pout. Finish with a dab of lipgloss on the fullest part of your lips.

14. Reach your ideal weight

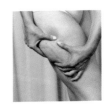

Cellulite is fat. So drop some pounds and you'll shift some cellulite.

But when a woman gains weight, the fat cells swell, and the fat effectively bulges out between the fibres in your connective tissues.

Here's an idea for you...

Want quick results? Try brushing shimmery bronzer on the backs of legs or thighs or smother thighs with a light-reflecting cream or lotion. They catch the light, making legs look smoother and draw attention away from the cellulitey bits.

When the fat bulges out between the fibres, the result is those dome shaped dimples we know as cellulite.

Fortunately, getting down to your ideal weight through diet and exercise means you'll shed the fat that causes cellulite.

Start by working out your BMI (body mass index). This is basically your weight in kg divided by your height in metres squared. So if you are 10stone 4lbs (65 kilos) and 5'4" (1.62m), your BMI is just under 25. (65 divided by (1.62 x 1.62) = 24.8) **If your BMI is more than 25, it's time to shift some fat.**

Start small. Make some changes to your diet, such as cutting down on your fat intake, and swap processed, refined carbs such as white bread and cakes for wholegrains. Start taking gentle exercise: aim for 30 minutes of aerobic exercise at least three times a week. Brisk walking is a good start.

Try these five golden rules today to kickstart your weight loss:

- Eat a healthy breakfast. Experts have found that dieters who eat a high fibre breakfast lose more weight than dieters who skip breakfast.

- Make sure you get your five portions of fruit and veg a day. Make them a priority before you eat anything else – you'll feel fuller already and will get more nutrients into your diet.

- Never say never to treats. Depriving yourself of your favourite foods often makes you want to rebel – and you can end up bingeing. Instead, just have a tiny amount and. Learn to savour instead of scoff.

- Eat snacks; yes honestly! Eating healthy snacks – fruit, pitta breads and hummous, nuts and yoghurt – helps keep your blood sugar levels steady. You'll never get hungry, so will be less likely to reach for cakes and chocolate. Aim to eat a low fat snack every two hours.

- Watch your portions: some people swear they eat healthily yet never lose weight. Huge portions may be the problem. You should be aiming for no more than a fistful of carbs and protein at one meal. But fill up with plenty of veggies.

Defining idea

'You are drunk Sir Winston, you are disgustingly drunk.'
'Yes Mrs Braddock, I am drunk. But you, Mrs Braddock are ugly and disgustingly fat. But tomorrow morning, I, Winston Churchill, will be sober.'
SIR WINSTON CHURCHILL

15. Great gnashers

Confidence, good looks and success are the kind of qualities a brilliant smile can impart. Dig out that floss today.

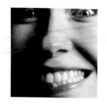

Imperfect teeth can make the seemingly beautiful less so. And a gorgeous set of pearlies can transform the merely plain into a radiant beauty. Having a pleasant smile makes you appear not just more attractive, but also more honest and trustworthy. And when you smile a beautiful smile, you make the person you're smiling at feel better and generate warmth, happiness and confidence.

White and even teeth, healthy pink gums and a convex smile are characteristics of youth. However, as the years go by, our teeth lose their luminosity and become dull, stained and chipped. A mouthful of fillings can also make your smile look dull and grinding your teeth can wear them down. So taking care of them and investing in the odd procedure (whitening, straightening, etc.) can actually take years off you.

To keep your teeth looking their best try the following:

Here's an idea for you...

Stained teeth? Try adding a drop of clove oil to your toothpaste before brushing your teeth to help brighten your smile.

■ Use a meticulous cleaning
routine and the best tooth
products you can. Brush your
teeth at least twice a day and
ideally after each meal.

Defining idea

'A smile is an inexpensive way to change your looks.'
CHARLES GORDY, author

■ Make sure you visit your dentist
regularly – at least every six months – and never miss a check
up.

■ If needs be invest in cosmetic procedures or braces.

■ Floss at least once a day.

■ Cut down on sugary snacks and try fruit, vegetables and calcium-
rich low-fat yoghurt instead. If you must eat something sweet
stick to chocolate, as with chewy sweets the sugar gets sloshed
around in your mouth for longer.

■ Finish meals with cheese, which helps neutralise the acid in
your mouth and prevent tooth decay. Cheese is rich in calcium
and phosphorous and this helps replace some of the minerals in
tooth enamel, thereby strengthening teeth.

■ Chew gum containing xylitol, which has been found to help
protect against – even reverse – tooth decay. It is also found
naturally in berries, mushrooms, lettuce and corn on the cob.

■ Avoid stain-causing culprits such as coffee, tea, cigarettes and red
wine.

Your teeth cleaning routine should last at least two minutes. First,
focus on the inner and outer surfaces of your teeth. Place your

toothbrush at a 45-degree angle and use gentle, short, tooth-wide strokes following your gum line. To clean the inside surfaces of front teeth, tilt your brush vertically and use gentle up-and-down strokes with the toe of your brush. Then move on to your chewing surfaces, holding your brush flat and brushing back and forth. Next, brush your tongue. Use a back-to-front sweeping method to remove food particles, which will also help freshen your mouth. Finally, gently brush the roof of the mouth.

16. Easy ways to lose a pound a week

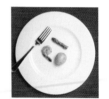

Mix and match these tips and you will look and feel slimmer with minimum effort.

One of the best solutions to losing a little bit of weight every week is to make changes that are so simple, you'll barely notice them. It's safe and possible to lose half a kilo (a pound) a week if you shave 500 calories per day from your food intake (or expend it through activity). Get started with the following clever little ideas:

- *Say no to crisps*. A regular 40 g bag has around 200 calories and 10 g of fat. So if you stopped having a bag each day at work, you'd save more than 500 calories a week.

Here's an idea for you...

Chew sugar-free gum or clean your teeth after a meal or a snack. As well as cleaning your teeth and giving you sweet breath, it sends you a psychological message that you have finished eating and that it is time to do something else.

- *Avoid large portions*. A large burger, fries and fizzy drink will easily stack up to 1000 calories, if not slightly more. Cut them out, or opt for the regular or small sizes which will cut the calories in half.

- *Watch what you drink*. Three 175 ml glasses of white wine will cost you nearly 400 calories. Three spritzers will be half that. A half pint of strong lager clocks up around 160 calories, while a half of ordinary strength is about 80 calories. A pina colada is easily 225 calories, while a vodka and slimline tonic is just 60.

- *On your bike*. An hour's cycling should take care of nearly 500 calories.

- *Sandwich swap*. If you have a little low fat salad cream in your lunchtime sandwich instead of lashings of butter, you could save up to 500 calories during your working week.

Defining idea

'Another good reducing exercise consists of placing both hands against the table edge and pushing back.'
ROBERT QUILLEN

- *Rethink your Saturday night take-away.* Choose chicken chow mein and boiled rice over sweet and sour chicken and fried rice, and save around 500 calories.

- *Walk more.* Walk to work, the shops or just for fun (but at a reasonably brisk pace) and burn up around 250 calories an hour.

- *Wash the car.* Wash it, polish it and vacuum it inside and you'll use up a few hundred calories,

- *Have a skinnier coffee.* Save yourself 170 calories by opting for a regular white coffee, made with skimmed milk, rather than a cappuccino made with full fat milk.

- *Party snacks.* Two tablespoons of tzatziki dip adds up to around 40 calories. Two tablespoons of taramasalata, however, is 130 calories. Thick meat pâté on French bread can cost you about 250 calories, whereas a small helping of smoked salmon on rye bread is a mere 130 calories. A cocktail sausage is around 70 calories. Wrap it in pastry and serve it as a sausage roll and you're looking at 200 calories.

17. Enhance your eyes

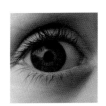

Easy-peasy eye care and make-up tips

Take off your eye make-up every night, keep dirty hankies or fingers away from them and pat – never rub – the skin surrounding them. Make sure you get lots of sleep, drink gallons of water, apply a regular dab of eye cream and treat yourself to the odd cucumber or teabag session. You'll also need a few good tools and clever make-up techniques. Try these:

■ Pluck any stray eyebrow hairs with a pair of tweezers.

■ Apply a pale or neutral colour over the upper eyelid, blending over the outer edges, to give a good matt base on which you can blend and build darker and stronger colours.

■ Apply a brown or grey eyeshadow, from the middle to the outer edge of the eye. Start with a tiny bit of colour and add more layers, blending as you go.

■ Brush a thin line of a darker shade along the upper lid. Add a little shading under the eye, too, at the outer edge.

■ Using white pencil along the

Here's an idea for you...

Bring out the colour of your eyes using contrasts. Pinks, mauves and greys look great on blue eyes. Or use really dark colours for striking contrasts. Avoid pinks if your eyes are red and tired; stick to neutrals or ivories instead. Remember: blend, blend, blend.

lower inner socket of your eyes can make them more striking. Dot a tiny spot of white shadow in the inner corners of your eyes to make them look further apart.

- If your eyes are small, you'll make them look even smaller by using eyeshadow or eyeliner around the entire eye as this will effectively close them up.

- False eyelashes can really open up the eyes. Try a few individual lashes on the outer corner of the eye, then add a few shorter ones, and alternate between the two as you work towards the middle of the eye.

- Eyelash curlers will help to open your eyes. Hold them so that your upper lashes lie between the two rims, then squeeze and roll upwards.

- Pop a layer of translucent loose powder underneath each eye to catch any of the eyeshadow that falls on your cheeks. You can then simply brush it away and won't have to reapply foundation.

- Stick to black mascara for drama, brown if you're very blonde or try the no make-up look, which is also more flattering against older skins.

- If you put mascara on the top lashes only and leave the bottom ones bare you'll look brighter and less tired.

- Use two layers of mascara for maximum drama, but don't let it dry between layers or it may cake and flake.

- Avoid putting powder underneath your eyes, as when it 'cakes' it shows up every crease and fine line and can be very ageing.

- Eyedrops are a great way to put a sparkle in your eye.

18. Sexy style

Image, style, look. Call it what you want, but you need to define your personal style.

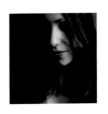

Style is something that should stay with you for ever; your own intangible look and image. There are three classic looks that work well – romantic (flowing skirts), flirtatious (tight, short) and erotic (gorgeous clinging fabrics, seriously grown up). Obviously the image you choose is determined by where you are going and what you're going to be doing. It would be daft to show up for a walk on the beach with your latest paramour wearing a leather skirt and stilettos. If it's a simple style you're after try a pretty floral dress, chinos and T-shirt, or a flowing skirt and a cashmere jumper, and go for soft colours such as beige, light blue or rose.

For a first date where there will be plenty of flirting going on, dress accordingly; a low-cut top or a short skirt (but never both together), go for warm, passionate

Here's an idea for you...

Transparent blouses are wonderfully sexy and it's possible to wear see-through without showing a thing. Fabric technology allows wispy fabrics that when you try them give just a hazy idea of what might be underneath. But if that's still too much, wear a jacket over it so there's only a glimpse of what's underneath. Alternatively a glimpse of lace works wonders.

Defining idea

'Penguins mate for life. Which doesn't exactly surprise me that much 'cause they all look alike – it's not like they're gonna meet a better looking penguin some day.'
ELLEN DEGENERES, comedian

colours like red, and remember your choice of underwear is crucial.

The vampy, flirtatious look is really not the one for a first date. You could come across as cheap and tarty, which he might think is ideal for that night but won't be any good for your long-term prospects. Unless of course you're just after a hugely erotic one-night stand, in which case, go for it. If you do want to dress in a way that guarantees he'll want to sleep with you then of course leather is good (preferably black), animal prints are also pretty effective, as are anything seriously short and figure hugging, lots of cleavage (if you don't have it, fake it), zips in strategic places and lace-up tops.

Remember you are in control of the image you want to project and the signals you want to send out to your date. Don't make them the wrong ones by either going over the top or showing up looking like a maiden aunt, though some men may even get off on that look. Best not to risk it though.

19. Feet first

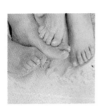

Attend to your feet daily instead of waiting for summer, when you'll find your work cut out for you.

The only thing separating most women and a serious Manolo habit is cashflow. But choosing the right shoe for the job can help minimise damage to the foot. When shopping for shoes, try to think first about heavy-duty wear. What will you be doing in those shoes? Walking to work? Rushing around shopping?

Specialists recommend we choose a low-heeled shoe (no higher than 4 cm) for everyday wear, with a rounded toe. We're also advised not to wear shoes for consecutive days because it takes shoes about 24 hours to dry out thoroughly; sweaty shoes cause smelly feet and fungal infections.

Wear high heels for a special occasion, by all means, but live in them and you'll damage your feet and cause postural problems. Moreover, they can shorten your calf muscles and make them look quite stocky.

Here's an idea for you...

Stimulate acupressure points on your feet. Stiff neck? Gently walk your thumb and fingers across the ball of your foot below your toes then around the base of your big toe. Aching back? Slowly walk your thumb down the inner edge of your foot following the bones along the arch.

Defining idea

'If high heels were so wonderful, men would be wearing them.'
SUE GRAFTON, writer

Wearing tight shoes can also cause bunions, curvatures in the toes and swollen, tender joints. It's worth assessing your shoe wardrobe, because wearing tight shoes can make the problem worse.

Regular foot maintenance makes sense and few treatments will make you feel more enlivened than a pedicure or a session with a chiropodist, so budget for a treatment once every three months. The rest of the time:

■ Regularly remove hard skin with a pumice stone.
■ Trim your toenails with proper nail clippers, cutting straight across and not down at the corners, which can cause ingrown nails.
■ Get into the habit of washing your feet each night with warm soapy water, but don't soak them for too long or too often in water that's too hot or you'll destroy the natural oils.
■ Stretch your feet and exercise your muscles by making big circles with your feet – clockwise and anticlockwise – and repeat four or five times each.
■ Make sure you dry your feet thoroughly, especially between the toes. Smother moisturising cream all over your feet, avoiding the area between the toes, and then apply some foot powder.
■ Treat your feet to a regular, soothing foot massage. You can either buy specialist foot products for this, use your favourite body cream or try essential aromatherapy oils diluted in carrier oil. Lovely.

20. Give it the brush-off

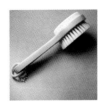

Daily skin brushing can help soften and smooth out orange-peel thighs in days.

You can skin brush every day in the comfort and privacy of your own home. It takes no more than five minutes of your time, a decent brush can cost as little as a fiver and you can usually see results within days.

Body brushing can help minimise cellulite by helping to remove surface dead cells, making the skin on your rear end look smoother and more even textured.

Dry skin brushing is also considered an effective way to stimulate circulation and boost lymphatic drainage. When these two body systems work optimally, your circulation delivers oxygen and important nutrients to your cells via blood, and the lymphatic

Here's an idea for you...

For a smoothing and circulation boosting bottom and thigh massage try this scrub. Mix 2 tablespoons of finely ground oatmeal together with one tablespoon of almond oil. Rub into the skin, then rinse off in the shower.

Defining idea

'The buttocks are the most aesthetically pleasing part of the body because they are non-functional...as near as the human form can ever come to abstract art.'
KENNETH TYNAN, theatre critic

drainage system removes the waste-products. When this flow of fluid slows down your limbs don't get much action and your skin in that region suffers.

Think of the skin cells that separate the fat cells in your bottom and thighs as bits of elastic. The more sedentary you are, the less nourished they become, and they become gradually thicker, and less elastic. As the fibres lose their elasticity, the fat that lies beneath them ends up bulging out between them, creating the dimples we know as cellulite. Some experts also believe skin brushing helps encourage new skin cells to regenerate and boost collagen production, which in turn helps elasticity.

Try it every day before your shower or bath and brush your skin in long strokes towards the heart.

How to body-brush:
- Start at your feet and brush your soles, toes and ankles and top of each foot gently but firmly with long sweeping movements. Brush the front and back of your lower legs, working towards your knees. Then rest your foot against the bath or a chair and brush from your knees to your upper legs and thighs, waist and buttocks using long smooth strokes. Repeat on both legs.

- Many women get cellulite on their upper arms, so don't neglect your upper body. Start at your wrist and brush your inner arm in upward strokes towards your elbow. Then brush the palm of your hand, then the outer side of your hand, and move up towards the back of your arm. Repeat on the other arm. Follow with gentle circular movements over your stomach and chest.
- Then shower or jump in the bath to remove the dead surface cells.

21. Sexual confidence

What is sexual confidence? And how do you get your hands on some?

So why do you want model looks? One reason might be to boost your sexual confidence. The un-politically correct truth is, if you're feeling lacklustre about your appearance it's very unlikely you're having a great sex life. If your lover loses stones and your love life is less than sparkling, you'd better start improving your bedroom skills because their sexual confidence is going to go sky high and when that happens, thrilling sex is never far away. With or without you.

On the other hand, if you've been feeling less like sex, ask yourself

Here's an idea for you...

Work on feeling more sexual every day. Think of yourself as a powerfully sexual person. Look for opportunities to make life more sensual. Flirt.

whether being 5 kg lighter would make a difference to your libido. If it would, then diet.

I would love to write with bravado that if you think having bigger/firmer/smaller boobs would improve your sex life you're frankly bonkers, but for some people it really can work. However, beware. Your goal is sexual confidence. If it's your partner who wants you to have surgery, you won't gain sexual confidence. And if you've had a boob job already, I very much doubt that having smoother thighs will make the difference. These are distractions, and your relationship with either your partner or yourself is at fault. Spend your money on therapy or a self-esteem course instead.

So what does work?

Change your perception. Do what it takes to feel as attractive as you can. Then start talking yourself up: 'I'm happy', 'I look great', 'I'm gorgeous'. Repeat your affirmations twenty times daily.

Look in a mirror. As we get older or busier, we spend less time looking in the mirror and try to pretend our body just isn't there. A mistake. Buy a full-length mirror. Look at yourself naked. Look at yourself dressed. Spend time preening. Throw out everything that doesn't make you feel great and look brilliant. If that leaves you with three items of clothing, so be it.

Spend as much time as you can naked. This reacquaints you with your body and puts you in touch with your sexual self.

Devote an hour a week to loving your body. If pampering isn't you, start exercising or go to a massage therapist or reflexologist. Anything that gets you back in touch with that thing you need for sex – your body.

Defining idea

'If you're one of those people who can't even look in the mirror naked, you need to get used to it...you're going to have to get comfortable in your own skin.'

DR PHIL MCGRAW, writing in O Magazine

22. Love the skin you're in

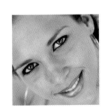

How to stay gorgeous during pregnancy.

The hormonal changes you experience during pregnancy can make some odd things happen to your skin, but there are simple remedies.

Facial spots

Oil (sebum) production increases during pregnancy, and this can make spots appear, particularly in the last trimester – a little like

Here's an idea for you...

Make yourself a gentle facial scrub from fine oatmeal from a health food shop mixed with honey and a little water. Smooth it onto your skin and make circular motions with your fingers before washing it off with cotton wool and tepid water. If you can bear it, splash your face with cold water to close your pores after you have finished. Avoid the use of harsh exfoliants.

they do before a period. Use gentle, hypoallergenic products to step up your skincare routine. Drink lots of water, and eat plenty of foods containing vitamin B6 such as wholegrain cereals and breads, potatoes, bananas and peanut butter. Vitamin B6 helps to control hormonally induced skin problems. Don't be tempted to take supplements unless you have consulted your doctor and *do not* take any of the anti-acne prescription drugs such as Accutane and Retin-A during pregnancy: they carry a high risk of causing birth defects.

Sweaty Betty

When you are pregnant, you sweat more. The weight gain can make you puffy in places. The upshot of this may be sweat rash under your boobs and in your groin. This is uncomfortable – and difficult to shift, once it occurs. Treat sweat rashes by bathing the area in cool water. You can also apply a sprinkling of cornflour to reduce chafing.

Itchy!

As your belly and breasts grow, and your skin stretches, you may feel generalised itching. Make your showers and baths warm rather than hot, only use mild soap or bath gel and use a moisturiser regularly (applying that could be a fun job for the boys). If your skin is really itchy, dissolve a cup of bicarbonate of soda in your bath for a soothing soak.

Stretch marks

Stretch marks are small tears made in response to the pulling and stretching your poor dermis undergoes as you expand. Sadly, the jury is still out as to whether any of the (expensive) lotions and potions available are effective. If it makes you feel better, have a go – you have nothing to lose, and it's a great excuse to make your partner give you a lovely rub down with shea butter. If you do get stretch marks, try not to worry. They start off red, but fade to silver.

Who's been painting on my belly?

You may wake up one day to find you have a dark line running from your pubes up to your belly button. No, your partner hasn't been busy with the magic markers; it's another of nature's little jokes. The line is called the linea nigra, found more often in women with darker skin and hair. It usually disappears again after the birth.

23. Bikini fit

Looking beautiful when wearing very little may require these clever tactics.

You can still wear a bikini if you have a less than model-like body. First, take a long look at your body in a full-length mirror. Assess your proportions and establish your body shape. Are you a pear, an apple, hour-glass, top-heavy, saddled with saddlebags or just plain, um, voluptuous? Decide which bits you'd like to hide and which bits you'd like to display with pride and then consult our tips.

■ *Flat- or small-chested?* Wear padded bras and tops with frilly details or horizontal stripes. Uunderwired bras with bows or flowers will add an extra dimension to an otherwise uneventful bustline.

Here's an idea for you...

Before splashing out on that gorgeous new bikini, make sure it fits comfortably and is also practical. Check that it does actually contain you and your curves when you're *moving* by running on the spot and raising your arms up and down. Also ensure the bottoms won't ride up uncomfortably by doing a few squats or kneeling down.

■ *Pear-shaped or big-bottomed?* Tie-sided briefs, are flattering on bigger hips. You can adjust them to fit perfectly and the ties detract from any lumps and bumps. Alternatively, choose bikinis with boyish shorts or flippy skirts.

■ *What about colour?* If you're trying to minimise a curvaceous bum and enhance a smaller bust, try a solid dark colour on the bottom and put the colour and pattern on top.

■ *Busty?* In order to draw attention away from your boobs to your face and at the same time lengthen your torso, go for V-neck swimsuits or bikinis. These will draw the eye from your décolletage downwards, effectively carving your bust in two. Another good tip to minimise a hefty bust is to choose thick shoulder straps.

■ *Big tummy?* Opt for vest tops with built-in support, which are great at covering a bulging tummy. Alternatively, go for high-cut bikini bottoms that come higher over your tummy.

Once you have it on

Think of the beach as an outdoor gym. Don't just lounge; get swimming, one of the best all-over body exercises as it works every major muscle group but is low-impact, putting no strain on your joints.

Wading through hip-height water is a great lower-body toner and can really help firm bottoms and thighs. And running across the sand barefoot is good for toning calf muscles, and will exfoliate your feet at the same time.

If you're feeling very comfortable in your bikini, a game of beach volleyball can burn up to about 300 calories in just thirty minutes and targets bums, thighs, pecs and wobbly arms.

24. Clean, green beauty queen!

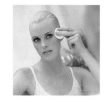

Cosmetics and toiletries are expensive so make your own!

The products we buy are cocktails of chemicals. Parabens and phthalates, which are potentially carcinogenic, are found in all manner of toiletries and cosmetics. We absorb substances through our skin, so it makes sense to make those substances as natural as possible.

Face
Honey, raw egg and oatmeal mixed together makes a lovely face mask. If you are having trouble with spots and blemishes add a drop of tea tree oil for its antiseptic properties – but be cautious when

using oils as they are very strong and can cause irritation if you use too much.

Natural yoghurt makes a good cleanser for all skin types, and jojoba oil makes a great moisturiser. Make a gentle facial scrub by mixing ground almonds, rose water, a couple of drops of rose oil and a few fresh finely chopped petals.

Hair

Camomile is well known as a rinse for bringing out highlights in blonde hair. Just make a strong 'tea' and use it as a last rinse after washing your hair. Rhubarb stems can be boiled and the liquor used to lighten hair. Wash your hair and comb through the liquid made by boiling a pint of water with two sticks of chopped rhubarb until it turns to mush, then straining it. Leave it in for half an hour and then rinse.

Sage 'tea' can be used as a final rinse for dark hair, and 1 teaspoon of cider vinegar added to final rinsing water is good for making any shade of hair silky. Raw eggs whisked in a jug make a strange but

Here's an idea for you...

Make your own bath bombs. Mix together: 1/4 cup baking soda, 1 tablespoon ascorbic acid, 1 tablespoon of borax powder (both from the chemist), and 2 tablespoons of icing sugar. Add 2 tablespoons of sweet almond oil, together with fragranced oil or herbs from your garden. Press the mixture firmly into moulds - cheap flexible rubber ice cube moulds are ideal. After a couple of hours these can be turned out onto waxed paper to dry for a few days. Store the 'bombs' in a closed container. To use them, drop them into your bath water.

Defining idea

'I'm tired of all this nonsense about beauty being only skin-deep. That's deep enough. What do you want, an adorable pancreas?'
JEAN KERR

effective conditioner for supple, shiny hair – just don't rinse with hot water or you'll end up covered in scrambled egg...

Bodies

Ground rock salt, or sugar make wonderful and invigorating body and foot scrubs. Add olive oil and a few drops of essential oil and a few fresh chopped herb leaves such as mint or lemon verbena. Just scrub and rinse for baby soft skin!

Baths

Simmer a handful of herbs or flowers in water for about 15 minutes. Leave the liquid to cool and sieve it before adding it to your bath.

25. Beauty sleep

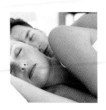

There's nothing more delicious and restorative than a good night's sleep. And here's how to track one down.

Vital repair work goes on when we're asleep and as we pass through its different stages, our skin gets replenished and cells regenerate. Lack of sleep will affect your immune system, making you more susceptible to infections, and can also cause us to put on weight since when we're tired our willpower is weakened and we're more likely to skip exercise and reach for fatty, sugary or salty foods.

Most of us need between six and eight hours, sleep to feel refreshed. Here are ten ways to a better night's sleep

Here's an idea for you...

Take a refreshing fifteen-minute power nap, ideally between 2pm and 4pm. when your body is primed for sleep. If you're at work find a quiet spot, close your eyes and focus on slowing your breathing and emptying your mind.

1. *Stick to a routine.* Go to bed and get up at the same time every day, including weekends, and if you must lie in, just allow yourself an extra hour.
2. *Try earplugs.* If you're woken in the middle of a sleep cycle by outside noise, you'll feel very sluggish. So if your partner or the neighbours are conspiring against you, just block them out.
3. *Try lavender.* Lavender has been scientifically proven to have a sedative effect on your brain. Try sprinkling some on a hanky, pillow or pyjamas.
4. *Eat for a good night's sleep.* Avoid rich food at night and wait two hours after a heavy meal before going to bed. Try a carb-rich snack before bedtime, such as some crackers or a piece of toast: carbohydrates release serotonin, which will help you feel relaxed.

Defining idea

'Tired nature's sweet restorer, balmy sleep!'
EDWARD YOUNG, 18th century poet

5. *Keep your bedroom for sleeping (or sex).* Never work, eat or watch television in bed.

6. *Sleep in the right position.* According to Chinese wisdom, the best position for restful sleep is on your right side, in a foetal position, with your legs slightly apart and your right arm resting in front of the pillow.

7. *Keep your bed fairly spartan.* Stick to crisp sheets and cool, loose pyjamas. Keep a window open if it's warm as a lower body temperature promotes sleep.

8. *Keep out of the wind.* If you're prone to bloating, avoid cruciferous vegetables such as cauliflower, cabbage and broccoli in the evening as they can make you too uncomfortable to sleep.

9. *Let go.* Keep a notepad by the bed for jotting down all those worries or additions to your to-do list that stop you dropping off.

10. *Relax.* Take slow, deep breaths in through your nostrils and out through your mouth and focus on your diaphragm as it moves up and down. Let go of each limb, each muscle, until your entire body is relaxed.

26. Yes, we have no pyjamas

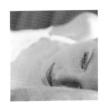

It's all very well working hard all day long to look sexy, but it's essential to keep up that image at night-time too.

When asked what she wore in bed, Marilyn Monroe replied, 'Chanel No 5'. I'm not suggesting you wear nothing in the middle of winter but there are ways to avoid looking like a furry toy.

The sort of thing you wear at night can define your image. If you go to bed dressed like a Playboy bunny, chances are you'll get treated like one. Now that even high street stores sell sexy nightwear there is no longer any excuse for you to get into bed looking like a maiden aunt. This applies even if you are sleeping alone – it'll help reinforce your self image as a sensual creature. Don't just give up and put on your grey (were once white) cotton jimjams. Think creatively, sexily and come up with something a little different.

You can buy all sorts of cute little night outfits. Short nighties for example, simple cuts with perhaps a ribbon or two, even if they're

Here's an idea for you...

When you are sleeping alone treat your hands and feet to a serious moisturising treatment. Put thick cream or oil on your feet and hands and massage well.

Defining idea

'As you make your bed, so you must lie upon it.'
LATE 15TH CENTURY FRENCH PROVERB

made of cotton are a good choice. I like those little French knickers and tops ensembles. They can be very simple, and really cute – understatedly sexy, especially if they're made from cotton. Please go for good quality though – polyester and other man-made fibres don't allow your skin to breathe, and while sweating is fine in bed, it should be from exertion not from simply overheating. Go for natural fibres such as cotton and silk, whatever design you choose. There is nothing more comfortable and warm than a pair of silk pyjamas. A good pair should last you forever and you can go to bed knowing you look great and will be snug as a bug.

You can also of course go for the Marilyn Monroe recipe and wear nothing but your favourite scent in bed. For this look you need to be smooth, soft and gorgeously clean or the effect will be lost. So wax, shave, whatever it is you do to stay stubble-free, then shower or bathe. An added bonus for soft skin is to exfoliate beforehand, preferably with exfoliating gloves. In fact if you do this three times a week you'll be amazed at the difference it makes. After exfoliating smother yourself with gorgeous smelling moisturising lotion or body oil. Similarly, don't overdo the scent, as there aren't many other smells in bed to detract from it. Try this trick: spray a cloud of it just in front of you and walk through it. You should come out the other end smelling just sweet enough.

27. Lighten up

Joie de vivre radiates outwards, which is why happy people are more attractive. Here's how to get your sparkle back.

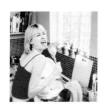

There's something appealing and uplifting about being around someone who's optimistic, bright and funny. A breezy, happy attitude and a good sense of humour can reduce stressful situations, diffuse tension, build bridges, heal relationships and make those around us feel happier too. So, it's little wonder that someone who makes us laugh or laughs with us is going to appear attractive.

A good laugh can reduce the levels of stress hormone in your blood by 30% and it can help burn calories (as many as 500 calories per hour). A strong wit can make a plain woman beautiful. The ability to tell jokes and make smart, witty asides will make you look both clever and confident, which is hugely seductive. Humour also enables you to laugh at your own foibles, find a funny side to embarrassing situations and find the silver lining to setbacks.

You don't have to be a laugh-a-minute comedian to have joie de

Here's an idea for you...

Get a sheet of paper and list your reasons to be happy. Start with today's events then cover life in general. Write down anything at all that puts a smile on your face or a warm glow in your belly such as a fantastic family, a great job or even a bargain pair of shoes.

69

Defining idea

'An inordinate passion for pleasure is the secret of remaining young.'
OSCAR WILDE

vivre. The key is to be able to have fun, be optimistic and see the best side of everything. A humorous attitude can help us to see life from a positive perspective and face problems with renewed ability and hope. And that's infectious.

If you've lost that sparkle, try these approaches:

- Spend time with children. They know how to have fun.
- Play games in the park, go to a theme park, have a girly tea party, that sort of thing.
- Look back at your last crisis. Can you find a funny side to it?
- Dig out old photos and look at the hairdos, guaranteed to put a smile on your face (well, everyone else's hairdo but yours will).
- Start savouring the pleasurable things in life. Try a new hobby, go on a shopping spree or get back to nature. Step out of your usual routine to find fun, laughter and adventure. Surround yourself with gorgeous things and your funniest friends.
- Get lots of fresh air. Run about, get soaked in a downpour, head for the coast and experience a sea storm, get up early and watch the sunrise, walk around barefoot, etc.
- Be your own therapist and try to write or retell your most painful or difficult moments with humour. Experts say this can be a good way to exorcise demons and flex those optimism muscles.

28. Cream's crackers

The effects may be temporary but adding moisture can smooth out cellulite to a degree.

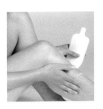

When your skin lacks moisture, it looks thinner, so those little pockets of fatty cells beneath the skin (which are the cellulite) are more noticeable. If you re-hydrate your skin, you reduce the appearance of cellulite. Aim to moisturise day and night – after a shower in the morning or after your bedtime bath. Expensive, delicious smelling unguents make it a more pleasurable task, but any good moisturiser or body oil will do the trick; you don't need one that makes special cellulite-banishing claims.

Another good tip to avoid dehydrating your skin is to avoid too hot water in your bath or shower as this can harm your body's lipids (natural fats). Don't soak for too long in hot water either. However sleepy or anxious you are to get between the sheets, make sure you do moisturise at night; experts say that's when the

Here's an idea for you...

Add avocados to your shopping list. They're full of mono-unsaturated fats and vitamin E, which are good for your skin. Eat them or make a moisturising beauty mask with them. Simply mush up two or three avocados into a soft paste and smother over your bottom – massaging it in using circular movements with the avocado stone. Then just wash it off with warm water.

Defining idea

'I love to put on lotion. Sometimes I'll watch TV and go into a lotion trance for an hour. I try to find brands that don't taste bad in case anyone wants to taste me.'
ANGELINA JOLIE

skin is more permeable so better able to absorb beneficial ingredients.

During dry weather or if you live in an air-conditioned or centrally heated room, try using a humidifier to put moisture back into the air. In winter put a bowl of water on a radiator.

Avoid over-using harsh soaps or detergent based cleansers or bubble baths; these can strip the natural oils from your skin and make it drier. Warm water is good enough to get your body clean unless you're really grubby. Glycerine is a good ingredient to look for in soaps as this is really moisturising.

The sun is cruel to cellulite sufferers precisely because it conspires to dry out the skin, which makes those orange peel dimples more noticeable. When you lounge on your chaise longue, baking yourself in the sun, dangerous UV rays release nasty free radicals, which attack the collagen in your skin. This reduces its elasticity. On your face, this spells wrinkles. On your bottom and thighs it means skin becomes more saggy, less firm and plump. Best advice, then, is to always use plenty of sunscreen (make sure it's minimum 15 factor). Reapply it often and stay out of the sun between 12 and 3 – the hottest part of the day. Or stick to fake tan, which is a great way to disguise cellulite.

29. Points on posture

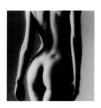

How you hold yourself can make you look and feel longer, leaner and more confident.

The key to great posture is to stabilise your core, i.e. the muscles that run around your body. Imagine there's a string pulling you up from the centre of your head. Whether you're walking, sitting or standing, think tall and 'feel' that string gently pulling you up. Your stomach should be pressed flat. Relax your shoulders down into your back. When they feel tight, raise them up to your ears, squeezing them up and together as hard as you can, then just drop them and feel the tension ease.

Position your pelvis as neutral as possible and keep your waist long. When you stand, make sure you soften your knees. If you lock your legs, you'll end up arching your back and throwing the rest of your body out of line. To avoid looking crooked make sure you put equal weight on each foot. Keep your chin parallel to the floor.

Sit at the end of your chair and slouch completely. Draw yourself up and accentuate the curve of your back as far as possible. Hold for a few seconds and then release the position slightly. This is a good sitting posture.

Here's an idea for you...

Counter bad posture with this exercise. Begin on all fours with your weight evenly distributed and your hands and knees shoulder-width apart. Pull your left knee towards your chest with your right hand, simultaneously curling your head towards your chest. Uncurl slowly, extending your left leg and right hand until they're horizontal to the floor; your back should be in a straight line. Repeat on the opposite side after placing your left knee and hand slightly forward of the starting position. Do five sequences.

Make sure your back is straight and your shoulders back. Your buttocks should touch the back of your chair. Distribute your body weight evenly on both hips. Bend your knees at a right angle, keeping them even with or slightly higher than your hips. Keep your feet flat on the floor. If necessary, use a footrest or stool.

Never cross your legs and avoid sitting in the same position for more than thirty minutes. Adjust your chair height and workstation so you can sit up close to your computer screen and tilt it up at you. Rest your elbows and arms on your chair or desk, relaxing your shoulders.

Strengthen those abs

Start on your hands and your knees. Whilst exhaling raise your right arm and left leg until they're level with your torso. Keep your hips even and look down so that your neck is aligned. Contract your abs, but don't tuck your pelvis under or arch your back. Pull in your pelvic floor muscles and pull your tummy button in towards your

backbone. Slowly return to the
start and then repeat on the other
side. Do two sets of eight
repetitions on each side.

Defining idea

'Beauty without grace is the hook
without the bait.'
RALPH WALDO EMERSON

30. Suck it out

**Here's what you need to know about
cosmetic surgery.**

If you want to be thinner surgery is not a good
alternative to eating less and being active, but if you have lost lots of
weight and the fat loss has left you with loose rolls of skin, a tummy
tuck might give you a confidence boost.

See several surgeons before committing yourself to a procedure and
ask them plenty of questions, including the following:

■ How often have you performed the procedure?
■ What kind of anaesthetic is used and who will administer it?
■ How long will the procedure take and how long will the results
   last?
■ Where will the incisions be and what level of scarring might I be
   left with?
■ What's the recovery time?

Here's an idea for you...

Try an instant image change with a haircut. Layers can make your face look slimmer as can highlights. Great hair works wonders.

■ Can I see 'before and after' pictures and testimonials from other patients?

One option for fat removal is liposuction, where a narrow metal tube is inserted into the fatty area via an incision in your skin. The surgeon moves the tube back and forth and sucks out the fat with a vacuum pump, leaving the nerves and blood vessels intact. There is a maximum amount of fat that can be removed from an area, so you might not be able to sculpt off as much as you like. It also doesn't affect cellulite and can leave skin loose. Following the procedure, your skin usually retracts and is bruised and uncomfortable. Healing can take a long time, with lumpiness and swelling taking up to six months to disappear. It's definitely not for the faint-hearted.

Neither is a tummy tuck (abdominoplasty). With this procedure, excess skin and fat can be removed and muscles tightened. There are mini, standard and extended versions. All leave a scar, from a low one at the level of the pubic hair to one that extends around to the back.

The latest high-tech techniques include LipoSelection by Vaser, which uses advanced ultrasound technology to separate out the fatty tissue from the rest before it is removed. This is claimed to be more precise, gentler and less painful, with a quicker recovery time. There is also the lower body lift, which pulls up all your slack skin around the hips, thighs and stomach. It is claimed to smooth out cellulite, flattening lumpy 'orange-peel' skin. You can also get arm and breast lifts, and just in case your hands don't match your newly slim and lifted body, there is now plenty that can be done, from getting rid of bulging veins to plumping up saggy hand skin with your very own recycled bottom fat!

Defining idea

'I was going to have cosmetic surgery until I noticed that the doctor's office was full of portraits by Picasso.'
RITA RUDNER

31. Quick fixes

Instant beautifiers for those hot date emergencies.

There are moments when we need to look super-gorgeous fast. Here are some troubleshooting tips to catch the beauty demons off guard.

Cover up those spots

First, clean the spot area using cotton wool and a medicated lotion. Next, apply a mattifying product or gel to the area to remove any excess oil and prevent your concealer from sliding off. Pick a concealer that's the same colour as your face, ideally dry in texture rather than creamy, and apply it right in the middle of the spot. Using a brush or your middle finger, wipe away any excess.

Instantly boost your complexion

Exfoliating to remove the layer of dead skin cells that dulls your complexion is the easiest way to brighten your skin and make you feel perkier. Splashing your face with cold water is a great pick-me-up, too. If you have longer, start by massaging in a rich oil-based cleanser and then remove it using a muslin cloth. Next, massage cleanser over your face and neck gently, applying deep pressure with the pads of your fingertips. Start behind the ears to stimulate the lymphatic system, relieve congestion and reduce fluid. Repeat this three times, then rinse the cloth, rub off the cleanser and splash your face with cold water.

Fix puffy eyes

Give yourself a mini lymphatic drainage massage to help beat the fluid retention. Tap your middle finger around your eye in circular movements, then lie down and place cotton wool pads soaked in witch hazel or rosewater over your eyes. Alternatively, try damp camomile teabags that have been cooled in the fridge. Drink plenty

Here's an idea for you...

For posh nails cut corners with press-on falsies. Pick the pre-glued ones and simply press them on over your natural nails. They should last up to three days.

of water too as dehydration can
make puffy eyes worse. As a long-
term solution, sleep with your head
raised higher than your body.

Brighten dark circles
Start in the corner of your eye and apply concealer a shade lighter
than your skin tone. Ideally, choose cream concealer as it's easier to
apply and goes on more evenly.

Tame frizziness
Use a leave-in conditioner before you blow-dry or add a few drops of
smoothing serum that contains panthenol or silicone-based
products to coat the cuticle and help it lie flat. Spritz your hair with
hairspray as it will help prevent moisture in humid air (which causes
your hair to frizz) from penetrating your hair.

Glam up your hair
Lightly spray your hair with water then add a root-lifting product to
give you instant body and volume. Start by blow-drying your roots,
lifting the hair upwards as you go. Then smooth your hair into style
using a natural bristle brush to give you extra shine. Finally, use your
fingers to tousle your hair into a dishevelled but glam style, spray
some perfume in the air and 'walk' into it. Instant gorgeousness.

32. The shock of the old

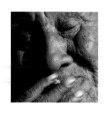

Growing older is part of life. Smoking gets you there quicker.

Seeing the impact smoking has on your face and body should give you the incentive to quit. Smoking ages its consumers. A recent research paper in *The Lancet* found that someone smoking a packet of twenty cigarettes a day for forty years had at sixty the body of a non-smoker aged sixty-seven and a half. The good news is that by quitting now you can move out of the aging fast lane and back in the middle lane, and start rubbing shoulders with smug, healthy women who know how to say no.

You might have seen those magazine articles that look at the effect a healthy lifestyle has on individuals. Often what is most striking is the illustrations which compare fit and unfit couples. By early middle age there is already a striking difference. The fit couple weigh less, and have better posture, skin, muscle tone and stamina. They

Here's an idea for you...

Ask people you don't know to tell you how old you are – the first number that occurs to them, not a figure to flatter you. You may be shocked to discover how many years the cigarettes have added.

look younger than the artist's impression of the other couple. If you think this is pushing the bounds of reality, take a look at a non-smoking sibling and ask yourself seriously whether they are wearing better than you are.

Defining idea

'My face looks like a wedding cake left out in the rain.'
W.H. AUDEN

Get a painful image of your future using a computer software tool like Photoshop. It's widely available, so if you don't have the program, there are sure to be plenty of people who'd be willing to take this project on for you. With a little imagination they can yellow your teeth, make your skin more flawed, and lighten and thin your hair. More advanced users will have no difficulty extending and deepening crow's feet, your frown and other tell-tell signs of aging. Print out and display in a prominent position.

In most large cities, shopping malls and tourist traps you can find an artist sitting behind an easel waiting to draw flattering portraits of eager sitters. Your purpose is to commission a portrait that adds a decade or two to how you look now. If the artist does not appear to understand, say that you want to see what you will look like in ten or twenty years' time. Take your picture home and frame it, having written in large capitals the words: STOPPING SMOKING WILL SLOW DOWN THE TIME IT TAKES TO GET TO THIS.

33. Back beauty

If you've never given your back a second thought, it's time to make up for the neglect.

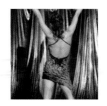

Disciplines such as swimming (backstroke), Pilates and yoga are fantastic routes to a long, slender back and shoulders. Also consider the Alexander Technique, a postural alignment method of adding inches to your height. Rowing is another excellent back firmer. Try this rowing-based exercise:

- Hook a resistance band up to a heavy object such as a table leg; attach it three quarters of the way down the leg towards the floor.
- Do a few stretches to warm up.
- Stand with your feet hip-width apart, a few feet away from the table. Bend your knees into a half squat with your hips behind you and lean forwards, keeping your back straight and your head in line with your spine.
- Take hold of the resistance band with both hands (palms facing). You should feel a stretch along the side of your body.
- Keeping your back, legs and hips in the same position, exhale and bend your arms to pull the band towards your ribcage, making sure your elbows stay close to your body. Then, gently return to the starting position, making sure you maintain the

tension in the band.

- Repeat the move fifteen times, building up to two sets of repetitions.
- Stretch afterwards.

Firm up your shoulders with this move. All you need is a light chair that you can pick up without straining. Aim for a set of six repetitions, three times a week.

- Stand with your feet hip-width apart and close to the chair. There should be a straight line from your ear to your shoulders, hips, knees and ankles.
- Breathing in, bend your knees and push your hips out behind you as if you're about to sit down. Keeping your arms shoulder-width apart, gently take hold of the sides of the chair. Focus your attention on the chair.
- As you breathe out, lift the chair to shoulder height, keeping your arms shoulder-width apart. Keep your shoulders down, your chin tucked in, your spine nice and long and your abs tight.

Tuck your pelvis slightly under and hold this position for three to five seconds without holding your breath.

Here's an idea for you...

Tense shoulders? Sore back? Try an aromatherapy bath. Add a few drops of Scotch pine, which is warming and good for sore muscles, or clary sage, which has anti-inflammatory properties.

Defining idea

'Good shoulders and a long waist are the most necessary when it comes to wearing clothes.'
OLEG CASSINI

■ Gently lower the chair and return to the starting position.

Keep your back clean by changing your towels and bedlinen at least twice a week and at least once a day. Slough off the dead skin cells that cause blocked pores and spots. Apply a good-quality cleanser using your fingertips, then remove it with a muslin cloth. Tea tree oil has good antibacterial action, so either dab some on the spots themselves or add six to ten drops to a warm bath and lie back in the water for up to ten minutes. Don't use it with soap, which can interfere with its healing properties.

34. The beautiful and the bad

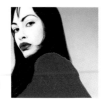

Top performers, models and stars probably feel more insecure than you do.

Beautiful women are held up as an ideal and yet top models, stars and performers suffer more than you think. They seem to have it all – looks, public adoration, money – but the cult of celebrity often makes people more insecure. Success is fleeting and many stars are anxious about losing their status or plagued with self-doubt.

Even the most beautiful women can have problems feeling

confident. Halle Berry is a former
Miss Teen All America, was the
runner-up to Miss USA and has
been voted into *People* magazine's
Most Beautiful People list nine
times: oh, and she's also an Oscar
winner. Despite all this, she
recently announced that she is very

Here's an idea for you...

Get some glamorous photographs taken
of you (if necessary by a professional)
and keep a few of them, framed, in
your bedroom. This is to remind you
that you are sexy, and the better the
photo the more confidence you'll feel.

insecure about both her physical appearance and her acting.
Knowing that such a successful, talented, good-looking woman is
plagued by self-doubts should convince you that beauty is skin deep.
There's no point in thinking that you would feel/be sexier if you
looked differently; confidence comes from within.

In *Madonna: An Intimate Biography*, J Randy Taraborrelli quotes dancer
Sallim Gauwloos who appeared in the movie *In Bed with Madonna*:
'She was very, very insecure…We would have parties, and there
would never be beautiful women invited. Only guys. She would
freak out if there was someone in the room more beautiful than
her.' Clearly, public persona and how stars really feel are two
different things – the grass is not greener on the other side.

Many women feel intimidated when they see airbrushed, perfect
images of women in the media. A recent survey in the UK found
only 3% of women were happy with their size; 25% of all women in

Defining idea

'A sex symbol becomes a thing. I hate being a thing.'
MARILYN MONROE

the UK are on a diet at any one time, although around half of them are not even clinically overweight. We are just obsessed with how we look, causing ourselves needless angst and provoking us to diet unneccessarily and fork out our hard-earned cash on products we don't really need, all in the hope of achieving something unachievable.

Once you realise that the real women behind these images of perfection are as insecure about their appearance as the rest of us it's much easier to stop worrying about your appearance and get on with your life.

35. Sex up your legs

How to slim, tone, smooth, soften and generally flatter them.

If your legs are carrying extra weight, you'll transform them by shifting some pounds with a low-fat, low-calorie diet. A combination of cardiovascular and resistance exercise is the best way to reduce overall body fat; aim for three thirty-minute cardio sessions such as running, rowing or cycling, and three total body-resistance workouts a week. You'll need to include dynamic work such as squats, lunges and step-ups in your resistance workout.

Try the following key exercises. Aim to do three sets of each exercise, three times a week.

- *Thigh, bum and calf firmer* Stand on a step and then take a large stride off it, extending one leg back behind you. Your front knee should be over your front ankle and the back leg should be long with a slight bend at the knee. Keep the back knee and heel off the floor. Contract through your tummy muscles as you lift yourself back up to a straight position. Change legs. Do twelve on each leg, building up to three sets.

- *Thigh toners* Stand with your feet wider than hip-width apart, with your toes and knees pointing out at forty-five degrees and your hands on your thighs. Pull up through your tummy muscles. Bend your knees, lowering your torso towards the floor. Keep the weight on your heels, and your spine in neutral position with your tailbone pointing down as you lower. Draw your weight onto one leg as you

Defining idea

'Darling, the legs aren't so beautiful, I just know what to do with them.'
MARLENE DIETRICH

drag the other towards it. Use your inner thighs to draw your legs together. Draw your legs apart and repeat on the other side. Repeat twelve to fifteen times on each leg, again building up to three sets.

Smooth and soft

For this you need to exfoliate regularly using a loofah, body brush or exfoliating mitt. Try body-brushing every morning before your shower or bath; use a brush with natural fibres and gently brush upwards towards the heart in long, sweeping motions. Exfoliators are great for softening the hard skin on knees too. Keep legs well moisturised at all times; creams and lotions help plump up the upper layer of skin and make it look softer, smoother and younger.

Bronzed

A tan will automatically give the impression of longer, slimmer, more even-textured legs. Fake tan is the best way to get a safe year-round tan. Always exfoliate first and massage in a light moisturiser before applying your tanning product. Don't overdo your heels or knees though, as these areas tend to get patchy.

36. A good dressing down

Learn the art of leaving something to the imagination.

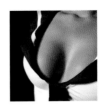

Sex appeal has a lot to do with confidence. So how does one dress confidently? The first thing is not to wear anything uncomfortable. It's very hard to look oh-so-cool if your bra-strap is digging into your ribs. Second, don't wear anything too risky. The skirt riding up to reveal a red G-string is not a classy look. I once wore one of those T-shirts with huge holes for the arms that were all the rage in the 80s. As I walked down the entire length of a double-decker bus to get off at Hyde Park Corner I noticed the whole, totally packed, bus staring at me. 'I must be looking particularly hot today,' I thought to myself. It wasn't until I got off the bus that I noticed the T-shirt was half-way across my chest. And in those days I didn't wear a bra. So safety first, wear stuff you know won't embarrass you.

You may be tempted to under-dress. And by that I mean wearing something so short it may as well

Here's an idea for you...

Go commando. Going out without wearing your underwear makes you feel amazingly sexy. And it's a secret only you know, until you decide to share it with your partner of course...

89

Defining idea

'Clothes maketh the man'
EARLY 15TH CENTURY PROVERB

not be there, thinking this looks sexy. Although men like a woman to be in touch with her inner tramp, most don't necessarily want the rest of the world to see their date looking like a lap dancer. The look you need to master is sexy but classy – chic and elegant with a hint of raunchy.

If your twenties have been and gone it is essential to avoid the mutton dressed as lamb look. If you are over 40, be proud of it. There is no reason why you can't be sexy, but think refined and subtle like Audrey Hepburn, and not Britney Spears. Have a model in mind when you shop. Before investing in those sequinned trousers ask yourself whether your icon would wear them.

The way clothes feel to the touch is also important, especially if you're aiming for body contact, so think about wearing clothes that follow the contours of your body and that are made of sensual fabrics such as silk, cashmere, velvet, mohair, chiffon and chenille.

There is such a lot of choice out there and the way you dress will make a huge difference to how you feel, how you sit in a chair, how you walk down the street ...and how sexy you'll be.

37. Creating curves

A dainty waist oozes sex appeal. Here's how to hone it, firm it and whittle it in weeks.

Studies show that waist-to-hip ratio – going in and out in all the right places – is a better gauge of a woman's attractiveness than the size of her breasts. To be precise, women with a 0.7 waist-to-hip ratio, i.e. waists that are 70% smaller than their hips are seen as more attractive. And that doesn't necessarily involve being thin! A small waist that curves into a generous hip equals fertility and youth – it's a sign that a woman has high levels of oestrogen and low levels of testosterone. In fact, in studies of IVF patients, women with a waist-to-hip ratio of more than 0.8 were less likely to conceive. What's tricky about waists is that their size is largely inherited; you're either an apple shape, an hourglass or a pear. However, the good news is that you can trim an inch or so from your waist by losing weight and doing some waist-whittling exercises.

Love handles won't simply disappear. You have to shed the fat first. Experts say that if your waist measures more than 81 cm (32-inches), you're overweight. If that's

Here's an idea for you...

Invest in a gorgeous corset. Anything that boosts your bust and cinches your waist will do wonders for your rating in the bedroom.

Defining idea

'The curve is more powerful than the sword.'
MAE WEST

the case you'll need to follow a low-fat, low-cal diet and do three to five sessions a week of cardio exercise such as running, dancing, cycling or power walking.

Waist-whittling exercises

Twist crunches Lie on your back with your knees bent, your feet flat on the floor and your fingers touching your ears. Contract your abdominal muscles and slowly lift your torso off the floor. When you can't lift any further, contract your side muscles and turn to the left. Then return your torso to the floor and repeat on the other side. Build up to three sets of ten on each side.

The bridge Adopt the press-up position, resting on your elbows. Pull your stomach muscles in tight towards your backbone, keeping your bottom down and your spine straight. Hold this position for as long as you can, being careful not to arch your back. To make it easier, drop to your knees. Keep looking down to the floor at all times. Build up to thirty seconds and repeat three to five times.

Horizontal side support Start by lying on your left side, resting on your left arm and with your legs extended outwards and your right foot on top of the left. Slowly lift your pelvis off the floor while supporting your weight on your left forearm and feet. Hold, keeping your other arm by your side, for ten to fifteen seconds without letting your pelvis drop down. Repeat five times on each side.

38. On The Shelf

Cellulite creams abound. But what works, what doesn't and what's really worth the money?

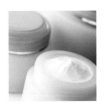

Cellulite creams alone, however impressive, aren't likely to transform fleshy saggy buttocks into a nectarine-firm bottom. Cellulite creams can hydrate your skin, so if your thighs and bottom have been neglected, rubbing on a cream will add moisture to the area and help plump up the skin. Many cellulite creams also contain temporary toning ingredients, which help improve skin texture; the effects can be pretty immediate but are temporary – good for a hot date, beach day, black dress occasion, that sort of thing. Longer lasting effects come down to a range of active ingredients:

Caffeine is thought to encourage the metabolism of fats, and help drain accumulated fluids in your fat cells, and boost your circulation. It is also toning.

Another key ingredient used in the more effective anti-cellulite creams is **retinol**. It's a derivative of vitamin A, which has been found to

Here's an idea for you...

Swap butter for low fat salad cream in your lunchtime sandwiches. Over a five-day working week you could save 700 calories and 12 g of fat!

Defining idea

'I will buy any cream, cosmetic, or elixir from a woman with a European accent.'
ERMA BOMBECK, humorist

increase skin renewal and boost the production of collagen, improving skin elasticity.

Another cellulite-busting ingredient is **aminophylline**, which is thought by some experts to enter the bloodstream and actually break down fat in the cells. One study found women using aminophylline cream lost as much as 8 mm from their thighs.

Exfoliating ingredients such as **AHAs (alpha hydroxy acids)** are often used in the latest cellulite-busting products. They're found in plants (citrus fruits and apples) and are used in skin products to help remove dead skin cells, thereby promoting the turnover of new cells. Thus far research has found the effects on cellulitey areas tend to be temporary, rather than permanent.

Natural ingredients

Most treatment creams are a combination of cutting edge technology alongside tried and trusted natural or herbal ingredients. Here are a few to look out for:

Gingko biloba: can stimulate your circulation and boost blood flow. A strong antioxidant, it may help slow down the aging process and help fight the free radicals that can cause your skin to age.

Gotu kola: This herb is thought to enhance the production of collagen. It's good for circulation and also has diuretic qualities and positive effects on skin tissue.

Guarana: a natural stimulant with a strong diuretic action, this seed is thought to help boost metabolism. It also has antioxidant qualities.

Horse chestnut: can help reduce water retention, boost circulation, and increase blood flow to the skin.

Butcher's broom: a plant extract with a diuretic action and which may help boost circulation.

Ivy: has been found to help boost the circulation. Its astringent properties may have a temporary toning effect on cellulite.

Marine extracts: carrageenan and alginic acid can help draw water into the skin which may help make cellulite look less obvious because it helps fill in the dimples.

Co-enzyme Q 10 is a powerful antioxidant thought to help beat cellulite by helping build collagen, and counter skin sagginess.

39. Hair care

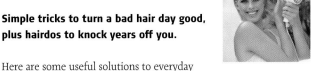

Simple tricks to turn a bad hair day good, plus hairdos to knock years off you.

Here are some useful solutions to everyday hair headaches. If you're really unhappy, it might be worth seeing a

Here's an idea for you...

Put your hair in a high ponytail and you'll look years younger. It will help lift your face and is flirty and cheerleader-youthful. A fringe can knock years off you too, and emphasise your cheekbones. And highlights around your face are anti-ageing as they lighten and brighten your complexion.

trichologist who can help with the likes of hair loss and solve difficult conundrums.

Book that trim

A regular trim – every six to eight weeks – really is the best way to keep your hair in tip-top condition.

The best blow-dry

Blot wet hair first with a towel. Spray some gel onto the roots and spread it evenly by rubbing with your fingers. Wait until your hair is almost dry before you blow-dry it and you'll do less damage.

For added volume, use a handful of mousse about the size of a golf ball. Also, try wrapping the top layers of your hair around two large Velcro rollers when your hair is 95% dry and then finish blow-drying.

Clip your hair up into sections. Start with the hair at the back of your head first, then the side sections. Pull each section taut with a large round brush and dry from the root to the tip. Use the nozzle to tuck the ends under or to lift hair from the roots for volume. After drying each section, give it a blast of cold air to help 'set' the hair.

When your hair is totally dry, part it. Now's the time to add a bit of serum to coarse, long or curly hair. Otherwise, wait until the hair is cool then spritz your hands with hairspray and rub it over your hair.

Defining idea

'I'm not offended by all the dumb-blonde jokes because I know that I'm not dumb. I also know I'm not blonde.'
DOLLY PARTON

Tips for curly or frizzy hair

Frizz is the result of too much heat, sun or chemicals used to bleach, colour, straighten or curl your hair. Choose conditioners with panthenol and silicone, which make the cuticle lie flat and make hair look smoother and sleeker. If you have naturally wiry or wispy hair invest in a deep-conditioning product. Never use too much conditioner even if your hair is thick. The right size for shoulder length hair is that of a ten pence piece, less if it's shorter.
Blot hair with a towel to absorb excess moisture. A wide-toothed comb can detangle curly hair without tearing it and help to eliminate frizz. Anything else can break or tear your hair, leaving it with split ends.

Apply a protective product before you blow-dry to prevent hair from dehydrating and then use a diffuser and your fingers to gently blow-dry. Avoid brushes or combs, as they'll just make your hair frizz. After drying, rub a few drops of serum into the palms of your hands then smooth it over your hair to calm wayward strands and seal in moisture.

40. Skin from within

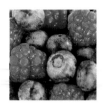

With great nutrition and a little care, you can achieve great-looking skin in no time at all.

You probably don't need me to tell you that fruit and vegetables are the main ingredients for a healthy, youthful skin. The antioxidants they contain mop up reactions caused by free radicals, created by such things as stress, pollution and certain foods. Free radicals can ultimately be the cause of degenerative diseases such as cancer and heart disease, not to mention premature aging (which is where your skin comes in). The main antioxidants are vitamins A, C and E together with the minerals selenium, manganese and zinc. Some B vitamins also have antioxidant properties together with some amino acids (building blocks for protein). Most of these substances can be found in a wholefood, fresh food diet. Berries and fruits and vegetables with red, purple and blue colouring are particularly good because they're stuffed with antioxidants and

Here's an idea for you...

Try to eat at least five portions of fruit and vegetables daily. And the more colours the better – try red peppers, yellow peppers, green peppers, red cabbage, sweet potatoes, etc. This way you can get enough antioxidants to help counter the effects of pollution. Be sure to buy organic though, as otherwise you could add to your toxic load!

contain a group of flavonoids called anthocyanidins, thought to be much more powerful than vitamin E. Antioxidants sometimes work together. For example, vitamins C and E work together – vitamin C allows vitamin E to be recycled in the body so that it can carry on working longer.

Defining idea

'All the beauty in the world, 'tis but skin deep.'
RALPH VENNING

Water your face daily

Drinking pure, fresh water flushes toxins through your system and hydrates cells carrying essential nutrients to every part of your body. Aim to *sip* about 2 litres (3.5 pints) daily. Don't overdo it though or you could end up flushing minerals out of your system, especially if you're gulping rather than sipping.

Fat face!

The other essential ingredients to healthy skin are essential fatty acids (EFAs). One group of EFAs is especially important: omega-3. EFAs work as a kind of waterproofer because they stop fluids escaping from your body's cells, keeping your skin plumped up and moisturised. Do an experiment – take a good quality fish oil supplement for three months (or flax seed if you're vegetarian) and note the quality of skin on the back of your hands. You'll notice that they're better moisturised!

You should also decrease the quantity of saturated and processed fats in your diet, as these compete with the good fats, making their job more difficult.

In general, the fresher the food and the more unprocessed it is, the wider the vitamin and mineral range and the more good it will do your skin!

41. Get the most out of your holiday

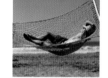

Maximum benefit with minimum effort.

While you're away make a conscious effort to

Here's an idea for you...

Eat like you're on a Caribbean holiday and spice up your home cooking by adding the herbs and spices used in exotic food. Spices also make a healthy alternative to salt. To name but a few, cinnamon, allspice and cloves provide antioxidants, ginger aids digestion and garlic boosts heart health.

eat better – lots of wholegrains, fruit, vegetables and proteins such as lean meat and fish. That way you'll be getting a wider range of vitamins and minerals. Whilst you're at it, why not make dining a whole a special experience? If you really relish what you're eating you'll eat less, as it takes twenty minutes for the brain to learn that you're full. The idea is to savour the smells, sensations and colours of the food, and to slow down to help digestion.

Also aim to drink more water. This shouldn't be hard as you'll want to stay cool poolside, but make sure you at least match every alcoholic drink with a glass of water.

Defining idea

'Come, woo me, woo me; for now I am in a holiday humour, and like enough to consent.'
SHAKESPEARE

Try to make time for breakfast, which boosts your metabolism and helps in weight loss. This shouldn't be difficult either as it should be such a treat to linger over breakfast, rather than having to run out to work with a piece of toast in your handbag.

There's nothing like a holiday somewhere exotic and/or romantic for firing up your passions. Use your holiday as a springboard for new beginnings. Now's the time to do the groundwork if you're thinking of making a career change, redecorating the spare room or suchlike. While you're on the beach, make a couple of to-do lists; things to do today, this month, this year, that you want to achieve before you're thirty/forty/married/infirm, whatever. Think back to old ambitions. Have they changed or have you neglected them? It's never too late to learn something new, see another continent, write your first novel, etc. The more fulfilled you are in life, the more confident and contented you'll appear – and 100% more attractive to boot!

Move that beach body

Aim to incorporate at least thirty minutes of strenuous activity into your day. Swim, try windsurfing or diving, run on the beach, play Frisbee – anything that gets your heart rate pumping. And use your holiday to strengthen your relationship and don't waste the extra time you have for talking, sightseeing, taking up new hobbies together or inspecting the hotel linen together. Get motivated!

42. Up in arms

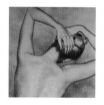

The rebellion against upper arm cellulite starts here. Yes, you can wear sleeveless dresses again.

Unfortunately, if you're prone to cellulite in this area you can't afford to carry excess baggage so losing those extra pounds is the first step.

Here's an idea for you...

Look for dresses with wispy chiffon sleeves – the sheer fabric will give your arms just enough camouflage but will still look glamorous and sexy.

The next thing to do is to really tone up your upper arms – it can take years off your overall appearance. Try swimming – both front crawl and breaststroke will help you trim down and sculpt upper arms. Both use powerful tricep movements, with pushing against the water adding resistance. Window cleaning is great exercise for the upper arms. If you do it once a week you'll get a good workout and have the cleanest windows in the street.

Defining idea

'Time may be a great healer, but it's a lousy beautician.'
ANONYMOUS

Best home exercise: tricep dips

The tricep dip is a simple exercise to tone up flabby skin on the underside of the arms and help diminish cellulite.

■ Sit on a dining chair, bench or even the side of bath, gripping the edge of the seat/bath or placing your palms flat down on the surface, close to your body.

■ Put your legs out in front with your feet flat on the floor – the further away your feet are the more you will work your triceps.

■ Using your arms to support yourself, ease your body forwards and drop your bottom almost to the floor, then return to your starting position.

■ Repeat between 10 and 20 times, rest and then do another 2–4 sets. It only takes a matter of minutes and the more you do the quicker the results.

Keep a set of hand weights or cans of beans next to the sofa. Every time you sit down to watch TV, use them to trim your triceps. Hold the weights as if you're placing them on top of your shoulders, with arms at right angles to your body and elbows pointing forward towards the TV. Lift the weights above your head and down again, repeating 10–20 times. Do as many sets as you can.

You may be able to improve the look of the back of cellulitey arms by self massage. Use some massage oil or good rich body lotion and use firm, circular movements and some gentle kneading.

Mesotherapy

Tiny pin-prick injections of a homeopathic medicine in your upper arms – mesotherapy – is also used to combat cellulite in this area, with some clinics recommending it as the most effective treatment for this part of the body. You will have to have a course of several teatments – usually one a week – followed by periodic maintenance sessions to prevent it returning.

43. Spa therapy

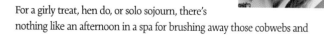

Spas are great when you want to feel like you're living the supermodel life.

For a girly treat, hen do, or solo sojourn, there's nothing like an afternoon in a spa for brushing away those cobwebs and making you feel all woman again. If you're new to spas, here are a few treatments/disciplines you may want to try – and what they can do for you:

Here's an idea for you...

Plan your own pamper party. Get the girls over, get into your dressing gowns, and experiment with make-up, nail colours, hair dos. Swap any unopened bottles of perfume or lipsticks that just aren't 'you'. You may find a few bargains. Add a few bottles of bubbly and some posh chocs and you'll be in heaven.

- *Acupuncture* An ancient Chinese therapy which involves placing tiny needles in certain points in the body – its channels of energy – to boost the flow of that energy (known as chi), in order to restore the body's balance and encourage the body to heal itself. Used to beat back and joint pain, digestive problems, skin disorders, anxiety and insomnia, depression, menstrual problems.

- *Reflexology* Diagnostic massage of the feet which uses acupoints to re-energise the body and encourage healing. The therapist gently manipulates points in your feet to treat areas of weakness. Wonderfully relaxing. Used to beat stress, anxiety, sleep disorders, back and neck pain, hormonal imbalances, digestive disorders, migraine.

- *Ayurveda* A 5,000-year-old Indian healing system which classifies you into either *vata*, *pitta* or *kapha* metabolic type. Treatment depends on your individual type, and usually includes various methods such as herbs, oils, dietary advice, yoga, massage, meditation. Often used for allergies, skin problems, digestive disorders, gynaecological complaints.

■ *La stone therapy* An ancient healing treatment, which involves heated and cool stones being placed along the spine, then gently massaged over the body to relax the tissues and soothe stresses and strains. Good for sore muscles, anxiety, neck and back pain.

■ *CACI* Dubbed the 'non-surgical face lift', this is said to firm the skin using the transmission of tiny electrical impulses and signals to stimulate muscle tone and enhance skin tissue. A course of ten sessions is usually recommended but just after one session you really can look brighter, fresher, less droopy!

■ *Oxygen facial* This involves the usual cleansing, firming and moisturising you get during a facial, and the smothering of lovely unguents. But the USP is the application of rejuvenating oxygen deep into the skin using a no-needle injection – or pressurised jet. Recommended to help boost elasticity and reduce fine lines, it's good for smokers' skin and acne, and results can be dramatic.

■ *Four hands massage* A sublime and very, er, thorough massage, administered by not one but two therapists using a combination of short, deep and long sweeping strokes to iron out those knots. Wonderfully synchronised, intense and pleasurable, and deeply relaxing. Great for sleep problems, sore muscles, anxiety, stress.

Defining idea

'*It is impossible to overdo luxury.*'
FRENCH PROVERB

44. The tan commandments

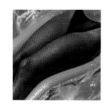

Having a tan makes you look thinner, healthier and sexier.

Preparing yourself for the suntan can take weeks of forward planning. You need to prepare your skin, especially if it's fair. Beta carotene supplements taken for a few weeks before you go on holiday can help you go brown. It can also be found in carrots and other brightly coloured vegetables. You should exfoliate with a body brush or exfoliating cream before you expose your skin to the sun. This removes dead skin and makes the tan more even. Once on holiday be sure to put on sunscreen about half an hour before you go outside. During the first few days, limit your tanning sessions to 20 minutes and avoid the sun between 12 and 3pm. Moisturise all the time, use a good after sun product in the evening and keep piling on that cream during the day. The sun drinks the moisture from your skin. It also removes collagen, the substance that gives your skin elasticity. So you need to make sure you have a good intake of vitamin C whilst on holiday as your

Here's an idea for you...

Try bleaching the body hair that you're holding onto before you start sunbathing. That way the hairs will be lovely and blonde, making you look even more tanned and gorgeous, and you won't be self conscious about them.

Defining idea

'Summertime and the livin' is easy.'
HEYWARD and GERSHWIN, American songwriters

body can't produce collagen without it. For the safer way to golden gorgeousness try fake tan. Products are improving all the time so if you purchase and apply wisely you should be able to avoid the dreaded streaks.

To ensure even colour remember to exfoliate before applying the fake tan and apply sparingly to areas like knees and elbows. Either wear special fake tanning gloves or wash the palms of your hands thoroughly immediately after applying.

You also need to prepare your body. This means eating sensibly and exercising at least two months before you plan to hit the beach.

Make sure you choose swimwear that suits your style. You can always wear the minuscule bikini while lying around trying to catch the rays but cover up with a sarong when you're wandering about. A classic swimming costume can be extremely elegant and sexy too: don't assume that in the beachwear stakes less is always more.

Sea water and sun can take their toll on your hair. Give it a deep conditioning treatment every time you wash it. Comb the conditioner through carefully and wrap your hair in a hot towel. If you're trying to go blonde then squeeze lemon juice into it for some natural and cheap highlights. But don't forget to condition it well every day as lemon juice has a drying effect.

45. Beauty A-Z

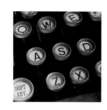

From the Alexander Technique to a zest for life, try these key beauty shortcuts.

Alexander Technique Good for improving your posture and relieving stress, muscle pain and injuries.

Balm Rub it on your lips, use it to tame eyebrows and smooth cuticles, and dab it over make-up to give your cheeks a lovely soft glow.

Vitamin C Great for skin and teeth, bones and gums – protects against aging by mopping up free radicals.

Dandelion tea A great diuretic that can help relieve bloating.

Eyebags Leave a couple of teaspoons in the fridge, put them over your eyes as you lie down for ten minutes and you've got a cheap and cheerful fix.

Fringes Make your eyes look much bigger, enhance all your features and take years off you.

Gels Anti-aging gels and serums are better for oily skin than creams, which can make your skin oilier and prone to breakouts.

Humidifiers A great way to keep skin hydrated if you're stuck in air-conditioned or central-heated rooms.

Indian head massage Age-old therapy based on Ayurveda. Reviving, relaxing and rejuvenating.

Juniper oil Stimulating and energising. Great for cellulite and as a skin tonic.

Defining idea

'Make the most of yourself, for that is all there is of you.'
RALPH WALDO EMERSON

Kumquats Rich in skin-friendly phytonutrients and bursting with vitamin C.

Lunges These exercises can tone up legs fast.

Mackerel Full of essential fatty acids (EFAs) which are good for your skin, eyes, brain and mood. Aim to eat three portions of oily fish a week.

Nails File them perpendicular to your fingers and square them off; it's the best way to keep them chip free.

Optimism Can boost your immune system, say scientists. Get more of it by listing ten good things that happened to you today.

Percale count The weave measurement on linen. The higher the count, the softer and better it is for your skin and sleep.

Quickie stain remover To remove stains on nails, dip them in lemon juice and then rub in some Vaseline to moisturise them.

Reiki A gentle touch massage; the practitioner lays their hands on you and you feel a lovely warm 'healing' heat move through your body.

Straight hair To make it ultra-sleek, blow-dry starting with the hair underneath and direct the heat along the length of the hair. When it's dry, smooth down with ceramic straightening irons and add a mist of glossing spray.

Tan Nothing slims, tones and lengthens like bronzed skin. Faking is safest.

UVA and UVB rays Damage and age skin and can lead to skin cancer.

Make sure you wear sunscreen at all times; nothing less than 15 SPF. Reapply regularly and use hair products with SPF protection to protect your hair too.

Veins Spider veins appear on the face and legs and worsen with age. Electrolysis, sclerotherapy or laser treatments are your options. Disguise them with concealer (applied after your foundation).

Writing Writing about your woes and worries can be an effective stressbuster and help reduce fatigue.

X chromosomes They make you female, so do something girly every day; try a face pack, buy some flowers, wear heels, go for cocktails with the girls. Treat yourself.

Yoga Your route to long, lean limbs and a balanced mind.

Zest Get more lemon in your life. It's a sunny cheerful colour, uplifting and warm. Lemons are tangy and full of the immune-boosting vitamin C.

46. Dieting danger

Everyone should be aware of the danger signs of eating habits that are out of control.

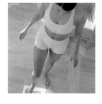

Eating disorders are difficult to understand, whether you're a sufferer or watching someone else suffer, but I think it is especially hard on the latter group. Why does someone who has starved themselves still insist they're fat? What is going on in the mind of someone who looks perfectly gorgeous yet steals away to the bathroom a few times a week to vomit? How can they be ashamed of what they've eaten and afraid to gain weight when they are obviously thin?

Some experts think there is a link between dieting and developing eating disorders, especially bulimia. The theory goes that dieting makes you hungry, which makes you binge, which then makes you feel guilty. In susceptible people, a purge (vomiting or using laxatives), helps to deal with the guilt and 'remove' the calories.

Millions of us diet without developing these kinds of illnesses. What has been discovered is that people who have eating disorders also share certain personality traits – they are perfectionists, who are eager to please, yet who have low self-esteem. When these factors are combined with family troubles (divorce, bereavement) or indeed certain family attitudes to weight and food, the spiral into illness can be quick. Ultimately, eating disorders are usually about control.

Check whether your own eating habits and attitudes, or those of a friend or family member, could indicate signs of disordered eating. If

Here's an idea for you...

Get yourself along to a self help group. Talking to others who have experienced the same issues and problems and can offer support and understanding without blaming you or making you feel guilty, can be a real help.

you're concerned, see your doctor, contact a self-help group or check The Eating Disorders Association at www.edauk.com.

Some common indications that issues exist or are beginning to develop include:

- Not eating in front of others, claiming to have just eaten.
- Being secretive around food.
- A strong fear of gaining weight, although you are an acceptable weight or even underweight.
- Distorted body image – believing you're fat when you're at an acceptable weight or underweight.
- Recurrent bingeing – eating too much in a short space of time, i.e. within a few hours.
- Shame and guilt after eating leading to using laxatives, or making yourself vomit.
- Obsession with exercise – working out several times a day for a couple of hours at a time.
- Judging yourself solely on looks.
- Ritualistic eating habits such as cutting food into tiny pieces.

Defining idea

'*It's important to remember that eating disorders are very complex conditions and are not about dieting going too far. The vast majority of people who diet don't have eating disorders.*'
LYNDEL COSTAIN, Diet Trials: How to Succeed at Dieting

47. Dress for success

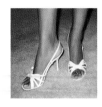

**First date impressions are extremely
important and the first communicator is
what we wear. So how do you get it right?**

You need to dress for the kind of man you want to appeal to, and for
the kind of relationship you want to establish.

Dressing to attract a man might sound like the past hundred years of
women's liberation never happened. But sexual attraction is an
important part of finding a partner and there is nothing wrong with
it: so get with the programme, have a good think about your best bits
and pieces, and get them out.

Here's an idea for you...

One quiet Saturday afternoon, try on
lots of clothes and find something that
is flattering, a little sexy and
comfortable; then hang it on the back
of the bedroom door as your SOS date
outfit, if you get panicked. If in doubt,
default to a little black dress. These
have served womankind well for a very
long time.

So how do you get the balance
between what you feel comfortable
in and what you think might attract
the right man? Firstly, you must feel
comfortable in whatever you wear,
as that will help radiate confidence
and an ease with your body. And
don't try anything frighteningly new
or too high fashion; lots of men

don't care that your shoes are the latest catwalk chic, but they might care if you take a head-first dive down the club steps because you haven't mastered the art of walking in them.

Defining idea

'Put even the plainest woman into a beautiful dress and unconsciously she will try to live up to it.'
LADY DUFF GORDON, 20s fashion designer

It never hurts to advertise, and men are basically visual creatures, so a glimpse of a taut thigh, a crisp white shirt with a flattering neckline or a well-turned ankle in some killer heels are all great tools in your armoury. However, there is a fine line between being tantalising and being tarty. This is where the 'one or the other' rule comes into play. If you have a great décolletage, feel free to hoist your boobs up and dab some seductive scent in pertinent places. However, you may want to team that stunning, sparkly, low-cut top with some simple flattering black trousers, rather than a denim skirt the size of a belt. Even if you also have fabulous legs, too much of a good thing can slide into slut. So choose one good area and work it to its best advantage.

Now consider where you are going. A miniskirt with a black polo neck is a winning combination if you have devastating legs, but not if you have to hide all your assets under the table during dinner. Be as objective as you can; you might love that skirt to bits, but if it's not going to work for you, put it back in the wardrobe.

48. Bottom's up

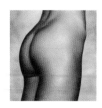

Having cellulite (as 85% of women do) doesn't mean you can't feel gorgeous. Try some bottom pampering today.

The truth is cellulite is just part of being a woman – nearly nine out of ten of us fall prey to it, including supermodels and Hollywood's A listers. That's not to say you have to embrace cellulite as part of your female-ness. But before you get stressed, depressed and obsessed about the cellulitey bits, take a moment here to get a perspective, and to celebrate your curves.

A friend's husband once took a mould of her behind, which was, refreshingly, generously proportioned. He gave it to her as an anniversary present – a wonderful pumpkin of a bottom cast in bronze. So first lesson is 'remember, men love curves'. In fact men particularly love fleshy bottoms when they're paired with a small waist.

Don't forget too, that your curves are there for a reason – legs, bottoms, thighs, tummies – they're all part of your healthy, functioning, living, breathing body. So think of a slightly dimply bottom as a sign of a rich, happy and fulfilling life. Oh, and a spongy bottom is also handy at weddings and on bikes; pews and saddles can be so uncomfortable.

So let's start by nipping that self-criticism in the bud. Time, instead, to celebrate that ass. Try some of these today:

Here's an idea for you...

Try this tiny bum-firming move you can do anywhere. Standing, raise one foot off the floor and kick it back behind you in tiny pulse-moves. Aim for 15 repetitions two or three times a day.

- Savour the good things about your bum and thighs – the excitement of slipping into new silky pants, that satisfying pain/exhilaration when you cycle up a hill, the sensation of rubbing lovely cream into your legs, someone else fondling your behind...

- Every day, promise yourself you'll do something that makes you feel good about your body – have something really delicious to eat, treat yourself to a day spa, go for a swim. Doing something pleasurable can make you feel happy.

- Stop buying clothes that don't fit which you're aiming to 'diet into'. They make you feel worse about your body. Instead, buy yourself something big but gorgeous that you can wear *now*.

- Make a mental list of your best bits – long, beautifully shaped fingernails, trim calves, firm boobs – stop focusing on your shortcomings and acknowledge your glories.

- Splash out on body treats: indulging really does boost your self-confidence – book a facial/manicure, buy new perfume, wallow in a luxurious, gorgeous smelling bath.

- Start taking some exercise. It can boost your mood, improve your complexion, help you focus and give you confidence in your body.

49. Short cuts to supermodel looks

The key to looking great is lots and lots of sleep, eating well, working out daily, good skin care etc. Surely there must be an easier way.

The problem is that you haven't quite found the time for all that healthy living stuff but what you do have is a date/party/wedding and just a few hours to get ready and you just have to shine.

First impressions do count, so make sure that you have all your necessary maintenance done for your special night out. It's not just the look itself, it's the fact that the psychological boost will leave you with a glow that shows. For a small investment that goes a long way, a manicure is a must. The cheat's way to a shiny head of hair is Aveda's Purefume Brilliant Spray On For Hair (www.aveda.com). This adds instant gloss and shine to even the dullest locks.

Defining idea

'Everything has its beauty, but not everyone sees it.'
CONFUCIUS

For a short-term skin solution you can't beat a facial. If you can afford the time and the money for a salon-based treat then do so – the more you spend, the better you'll feel.

However, if you can't, there's plenty you can do at home. Forget cucumber slices on the eyes – it'll make you feel too much like a distressed divorcee and not enough like a sex kitten. Instead go for the likes of Origins 'Clear Improvement' (www.origins.com), which is a black charcoal mask to draw out pore-clogging impurities, followed by an Elemis 'Fruit Active Rejuvenating Mask' (www.elemis.com).

Here's an idea for you...

The gruesome fact is that 'pants of steel' (as India Knight puts it) are the short-term solution to waistline emergencies. On this one, it's only right to go with the advice of India Knight herself and get yourself the ultimate pair – Nancy Ganz Bodyslimmers Hi Waisted Belly Buster.

Remember to have a hot bath before you go out to plump out your complexion with all that steam and to get the circulation going so that you appear rosy and, therefore, healthy.

For an energy boost try supergreens. These are ground up superfoods – extremely health promoting vegetables, algae and sprouted grasses – which give a shot of optimum nutrition in one glass. Upside: you'll swear you can actually notice the difference in energy levels and well-being. Downside: they tend to taste disgusting. So, mix these life-giving powders with a little juice and down the hatch. Two that taste just about OK and give you a spring in your step are Kiki's Nature's Living Superfood (www.kiki-health.co.uk) and Perfect Food by Garden of Life (www.gardenoflifeusa.com).

Defining idea

'Grace in women has more effect than beauty.'
WILLIAM HAZLITT

Some people also recommend performing a couple of press-ups to flush the blood through your system and bring a healthy glow to your skin. (Not so many that you arrive out of breath and beetroot faced.) Before you make your entrance, try spritzing your face with a water spray, which helps cool you down and also freshens up your make-up – so carry your own supply with you at all times.

50. Beauty and the breast

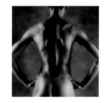

The old adage that men like something they can get hold of still holds true.

The fact that Marilyn Monroe was a size 14 has often been quoted. The first time I heard it I couldn't believe it. I thought it was impossible that a sex symbol could be so, well, large. In fact if you watch her wiggling down the platform in the film Some Like it Hot, you can see she really does have what you might call child-bearing hips. Yet she is one of the sexiest film stars of all time.

So, if you've got it, flaunt it. If you are voluptuous, use it, play to your advantages. Wear clothes that accentuate your chest and hips, thus making your waist look thinner. Wear tops that accentuate your cleavage and wear bras that make the best of your breasts. If you are short then avoid horizontal stripes as they will accentuate your size; go for vertical stripes or plain colours. Choose clothes and colours that exaggerate your femininity; long flowing dresses, pastel colours, lace (with a hint of cleavage showing of course). If you worry about your bottom being too big, wear loose trousers with side fastenings. These flatten your tummy and minimise your bum.

Here's an idea for you...

If you are toned you will never look out of shape, no matter how voluptuous you are. You should do sit-ups, press-ups and bottom clenches every day. Hone those beautiful curves until they are irresistibly perfect.

The skinny ideal that we're all supposed to aspire to is only something propagated by fashion designers and marketing forces, whereas the hourglass or pear-shaped female form has been idolised for centuries.

Fewer than 3 per cent of American women are the size of the models that grace the front covers of all the magazines. So 97 per cent of them are unattractive, right? That means an awful lot of so-called unattractive women are getting married, laid, falling in love, having

Defining idea

'I know that there are nights when I have power. When I put on something and walk in somewhere and if there is a man who doesn't look at me, it's because he's gay.'
KATHLEEN TURNER, actor

children every day. Go figure. It's got to be the magazines that have got it wrong.

The other good news is that being slightly plump makes you look younger. Skinny women have more lines. As she grows older a woman has to make a choice between her face and her bum. She can't keep both in the same condition as when she was 20. For that reason, some beauty experts recommend that women over 35 should not try to lose weight.

51. Let's face facts

Skin is your body's biggest organ. It mirrors your inner health and, unlike your other organs, the world gets to look at it.

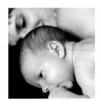

You can do much to improve your skin from both the outside and inside.

There are some real health benefits to be had from being in sunshine, but like everything you can have too much of a good thing. Sunshine is dehydrating, as hot sun will increase the evaporation of water from the surface of the skin. You need plenty of antioxidants or agents that protect us against harmful environmental factors. These can be found in, you guessed it, fruit and vegetables. Obviously, plenty of water is the order of the day too – at least 2 litres (3.5 pints) of the stuff. And knock off the cigarettes and the alcohol! You know it's bad for you and it's really not helping your body's detoxification pathways (your liver in particular). One last nag, remember to incorporate lots of essential fatty acids in your diet as your skin needs to be well oiled, so include lots of nuts, seeds and oily fish in your diet.

Here's an idea for you...

Treat yourself to a salon facial massage – they're wonderful for the circulation. Alternatively do it yourself with a home massage – the rose facial oil from Neal's Yard (www.nealsyardremedies.com) is especially good.

Routine, routine!

You don't have to spend a fortune on skincare, and expensive doesn't always equal good, but getting into a routine is vital. Always take your make-up off, however late you get to bed! Make-up is essentially dirt to your skin so if you leave it on all night it'll clog up pores and leave you with spotty skin.

The most important thing you can do to perk your skin up is to exfoliate. Exfoliation isn't something you need to do every day – once a week should be fine. As we get older, we really need to make sure we're exfoliating on a really regular basis otherwise if we don't clear out the dead cells, wrinkles can look deeper. Older skin too needs a gentler

touch when it comes to exfoliation –
no pulling and rubbing or harsh
products like creams based on fruit
acids. Fresh (www.fresh.com) have a
really wonderful facial scrub that is
moisturising at the same time.
Alternatively, make your own
exfoliator with 2 teaspoons of fine
oatmeal and 2 teaspoons of ground
almonds with some rose water to
blend. Rub it in small circular motions over your skin, then rinse off.

52. Fashionista freebie

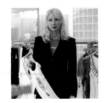

How can we dress beyond our means?

If you have fashionista aspirations but burger-flipper finances, then
you're going to have to adopt some different tactics if you want to doll
yourself up at knock-down prices.

If you're going to be photographed and that photograph is going to be
published then you are an immediate billboard. While you might not

get the front cover of Heat there are local suppliers for whom the middle pages of the local newspaper are realistically just as interesting. Give it a bit of thought and then try calling a small designer who might want to get noticed. Make it crystal clear that you are asking to borrow the items just for that one event, and that you are taking responsibility for cleaning/damage etc.

Here's an idea for you...

Many people swear by the charity shops for designer labels. The trick is to find those in the right kind of areas where people dispose of clothes because they are last season rather than scruffy. Hence, rootling around the Oxfam shop in Chelsea, for example, is more likely to bring results than grubbing through the racks in Grungeness.

Slightly further down the slippery moral slope is the much used but little talked of tactic of abusing the shops' return policy. Fewer and fewer shops will give you your money back these days if you return an item, but even those that don't will give you an exchange for the full value. If you're shameless enough this means you can effectively use them as a lending library for fashion, returning an item the next day and redeeming it against the next in your wish list. Do remember to check the returns policy of the shop, to keep the receipt, and don't forget that if someone at the soiree spills red wine on you, then congratulations, you just bought it.

A slightly less dodgy way of making your hard-earned diva dollars go further is to join a real lending library of to-die-for divaware. If you want to be seen with the most luscious handbag, for example, sign up to 'Be A

Defining idea

'Fashion is not frivolous. It is a part of being alive today.'
MARY QUANT

Fashionista' at www.be-a-fashionista.co.uk. For a fee you join up and you are then free to pick a handbag from a range of designer must-haves, which you use for as long as you like. When you fancy another, or simply can't be seen dead with the same one (daahhling), then you swap it for a different one from the selection. There are three different levels of membership, depending on the exclusivity of the bags you're after. The choice starts with 'Diva In Training' from less than £30 a month. For that you get the likes of Antik Batik or Jamin Puech. Moving up in the world you can join the 'Style Guru' level (Prada, Fendi) or splash out for the full-on 'Fashionista' class (nearly £100 a month) and prance around with Marc Jacobs, Dolce & Gabbana or Luella.